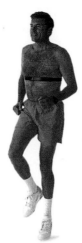

Health And Healing
The Natural Way

A Healthy Heart

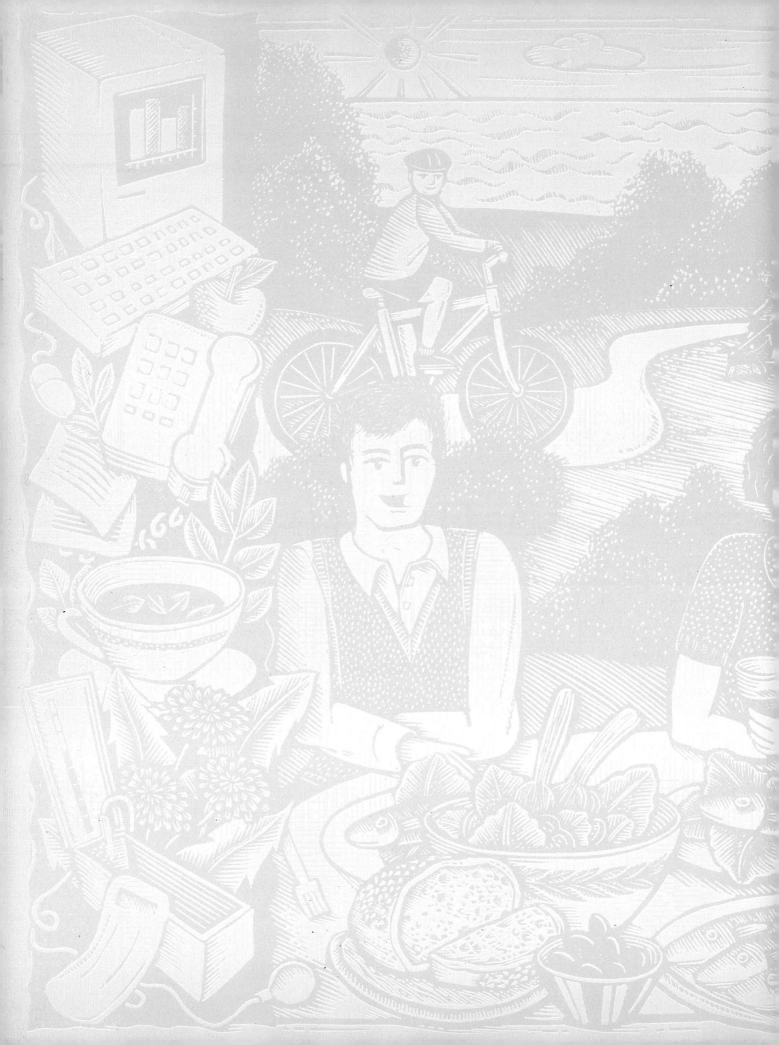

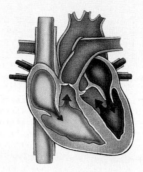

HEALTH AND HEALING
THE NATURAL WAY

A HEALTHY HEART

Reader's
Digest

PUBLISHED BY

THE READER'S DIGEST ASSOCIATION, INC.

PLEASANTVILLE, NEW YORK / MONTREAL

A READER'S DIGEST BOOK
Produced by
Carroll & Brown Limited, London

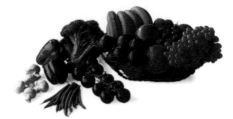

CARROLL & BROWN

Managing Editor Denis Kennedy
Art Director Chrissie Lloyd

Series Editor Arlene Sobel
Series Art Editor Johnny Pau

Editor Sharon Freed

Assistant Editor Laura Price

Art Editor Louisa Cameron
Designer Helen George

Photographers Ian Boddy, David Murray

Production Lorraine Baird, Wendy Rogers,
Amanda Mackie

Computer Management John Clifford, Caroline Turner

The acknowledgments and credits that appear on page 160
are hereby made a part of this copyright page.

Library of Congress Cataloging in Publication Data

A healthy heart / Reader's Digest.
   p. cm. -- (Health and healing the natural way)
   Includes index.
   ISBN 0-7621-0263-2
   1. Heart--Popular works. 2. Heart--Diseases--Prevention.
I. Reader's Digest Association. II. Series.

RC672 .H38 2000   99-054731
616.1'205–dc21

The information in this book is for reference only;
it is not intended as a substitute for a doctor's diagnosis and care.
The editors urge anyone with continuing medical problems
or symptoms to consult a doctor.

CONSULTANTS

Professor A.J. Camm QHP, MD, FRCP, FESC, FACC, CStJ
Department of Cardiological Sciences
St. George's Hospital, London

Lucille Daniels BSc (Nutrition)
State Registered Dietician

Susanna Dowie LicAc, MTAcS, RWTA
Licentiate in Acupuncture and Chinese Medicine
Member of the Traditional Acupuncture Society

Dr. Lesley Hickin MB, BS, BSc, DRCOG, MRCGP
General Practitioner

Roger Newman Turner BAc, ND, DO
Member of the Register of Naturopaths
Member of the Register of Osteopaths

Bob Smith

MEDICAL ILLUSTRATIONS CONSULTANT

Dr. Frances Williams MB, BChir, MRCP, DTM&H

CONTRIBUTORS

May Winnifred Annexton, Anita Bean BSc,
Ellen Dupont, Richard Emerson, Elaine Harbige,
Nigel Howard, Sharon Talbot, Stephen Ulph

FOR THE READER'S DIGEST

Series Editor Gayla Visalli

READER'S DIGEST ILLUSTRATED REFERENCE BOOKS, U.S.

Editor in Chief, Christopher Cavanagh
Editorial Director, health & medicine Wayne Kalyn
Design Director, health & medicine Barbara Rietschel

READER'S DIGEST BOOKS & HOME ENTERTAINMENT, CANADA

Vice President and Editorial Director Deirdre Gilbert
Managing Editor Philomena Rutherford
Art Director John McGuffie

Address any comments about *A Healthy Heart* to Editor in Chief,
U.S. Illustrated Reference Books, Pleasantville, NY 10570

A HEALTHY HEART

More and more people today are choosing to take greater responsibility for their own health care rather than relying on a doctor to step in with a cure when something goes wrong. We now recognize that we can influence our health by making improvements in lifestyle, such as a maintaining a better diet, doing more exercise, and reducing stress. People are also becoming increasingly aware that there are other healing methods—some new, others ancient—that can help to prevent illness or be used as a complement to orthodox medicine.

The series *Health and Healing the Natural Way* will help you to make informed choices by giving you clear, comprehensive, straightforward, and encouraging information and advice about methods of improving your health. The series explains the many different natural therapies now available, including aromatherapy, herbalism, acupressure, and a number of others, and the circumstances in which they may be of benefit when used in conjunction with conventional medicine.

The approach of *A HEALTHY HEART* reflects the idea that a healthy person is one whose mind and body work in concert to achieve that goal. Throughout the following pages the message you will see time and again is that the responsibility for a healthy heart is in your own hands. The well-being of the heart should be a major concern for everyone because without a well-functioning heart, the quality of human life is significantly reduced.

It is vital to understand the underlying causes of heart disease so that you can keep your heart functioning at its maximum capacity. Keeping your heart strong and helping it to recover from heart disease or a heart attack may mean changing your behavior, habits, and even some aspects of your personality. Throughout the book natural therapies are suggested for maintaining and helping to restore the health of your heart, and the book shows you how these therapies can be used alongside orthodox medicine for the greatest benefit.

CONTENTS

INTRODUCTION: YOU AND YOUR HEART *8*

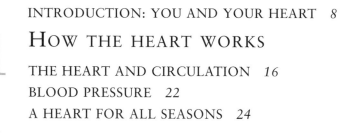

1 HOW THE HEART WORKS

THE HEART AND CIRCULATION *16*

BLOOD PRESSURE *22*

A HEART FOR ALL SEASONS *24*

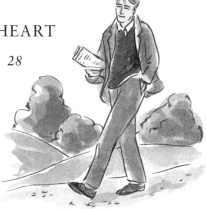

2 LIFESTYLE AND A HEALTHY HEART

WHO IS AT RISK FOR HEART DISEASE? *28*

A postmenopausal woman 30

AVOIDING HEART DISEASE *34*

Helpful ways to quit smoking 36

Autogenic training 42

THE IMPORTANCE OF CHECKUPS *44*

A middle-aged woman at risk 45

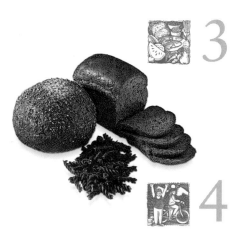

3 EATING TO PROTECT YOUR HEART

DIET AND HEART DISEASE *48*

A gourmet traveler 50

FATS AND HEART DISEASE *52*

FOODS FOR A HEALTHY HEART *58*

Reducing your risk with the heart diet 62

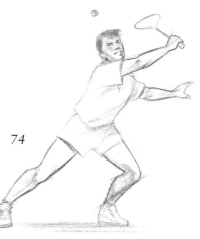

4 EXERCISING TO PROTECT YOUR HEART

EXERCISE AND YOUR HEART *66*

The personal trainer 72

MAKING EXERCISE PART OF YOUR LIFE *74*

An angina sufferer 77

Improving your flexibility with stretching 78

Getting in shape with toning 80

THE ART OF RELAXATION *82*

5

DIAGNOSIS AND TREATMENT OPTIONS

SIGNS AND SYMPTOMS *86*

DIAGNOSTIC TESTS *90*

An airline pilot at risk 92

Monitoring your heart with home tests 96

NATURAL TREATMENT OPTIONS *99*

6

HEART AND CIRCULATORY DISORDERS

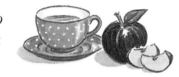

HEART DISORDERS *106*

A child with a hole in the heart 109

Cardiopulmonary resuscitation 116

The naturopath 122

CIRCULATORY DISORDERS *124*

7

THE ROAD TO RECOVERY

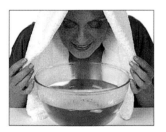

SPEEDING YOUR RECOVERY *132*

A recovering cardiac case 134

Rehabilitation manager 138

CONTROLLING BLOOD PRESSURE *140*

CHANGING YOUR EATING HABITS *142*

Feldenkrais Method 144

MANAGING STRESS *146*

*Helping your heart with stress
reduction 150*

CONTROLLING ANGER
AND HOSTILITY *152*

An angry man 154

INDEX *157*

ACKNOWLEDGMENTS *160*

YOU AND YOUR HEART

Modern life is setting your heart a tough challenge. How you treat this vital organ will determine your health now and in the future.

THE MYTHICAL HEART
For centuries the heart has been deemed the seat of our emotions. In this 16th-century painting, the heart is shown connected with the feeling of love.

THE HEALTHY HEART DIET
Eating at least five servings of fruits and vegetables every day provides antioxidants that help fight disease. They also provide fiber (as do whole-grain cereal products), which helps lower cholesterol levels and keep the heart arteries from becoming clogged with fatty plaque.

Few people need to be reminded of the crucial role played in the body by the heart. Unlike most other organs, the heart makes its presence palpably felt in one way or another every day. Its dramatic leap into pulsating life in response to feelings of attraction, excitement, alarm, and the whole spectrum of human emotion has always aroused interest and wonder, and the mystery of its action has secured for it a privileged place in the folklore, mythology, and language of men and women the world over.

Although anatomical study has long since ousted the heart from its former position as the conscience and center of a person's being, modern medical research is now bringing to light the sensitivity of the heart to such factors as exercise, diet, habits, and personality, so we are now able to take fuller responsibility for its health. Because the heart is an involuntary muscle, working without our conscious effort, most people tend to take its proper functioning for granted until something goes amiss. They don't realize how much influence they can have on its health.

Statistics show that heart problems are now occurring with an alarming frequency. This century has seen a massive increase in the number of people suffering from degenerative heart disease, which is now the biggest cause of death and disability in the Western world. In North America it kills as many people as all other diseases put together, including cancer, and as many as one in five of the population suffer from high blood pressure—a poor prognosis for the heart's health. In America more than 800,000 people die from heart attacks and other heart conditions, such as congestive failure, every year. The American Heart Association estimates that more than 60 million Americans have some form of cardiovascular disease. And in Canada some 76,000 men and women die from coronary heart and artery disease annually.

Many people associate problems related to the functioning of the heart with the onset of middle age. But there is nothing inevitable about heart disease. It is not necessarily a natural product of old age or decline. It can result from a lifetime of bad habits and diet, in which case it is largely self-inflicted and avoidable. The tragic fact is that heart disease is striking people down in the prime of their lives.

THE CAUSES OF HEART DISEASE

The heart is the pump at the center of the body's plumbing system, the transportation network of tubes that supplies blood to all parts of the body. Along with input from the brain and nervous system, the heart regulates the rate at which blood is pumped to the various organs, as well as the amount of blood that is needed in different situations, such as exercise or stress. Even a minor defect in the heart or its arteries can cause major symptoms and problems.

In some cases the heart may be defective at birth or sustain damage to the valves as a result of rheumatic fever or another infectious illness. When the heart muscle is damaged by illness or such factors as alcoholism, heart failure may occur. But in the vast majority of cases, heart disease is actually the end result of the gradual deterioration of the coronary arteries.

In the Western world we eat too much (often of the wrong things), drink too much alcohol, smoke too much tobacco, exercise too little, and live in unhealthy environments. All these things contribute to damage of the blood vessels. When they become constricted with a buildup of fatty plaque, the heart has to work harder to maintain the all-important free flow of blood and is consequently put under strain. A heart attack is simply a case of the pump or a connecting pipe giving up when the odds are stacked against it.

MODERN MEDICINE

Today there are ingenious and sophisticated methods for diagnosing heart and circulatory ailments. These range from a simple physical examination (taking the pulse and blood pressure and listening to the heart with a stethoscope), to an electrocardiogram (ECG) and exercise stress test, to the more complex scans and such invasive procedures as cardiac catheterization and coronary

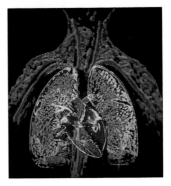

POSITION OF THE HEART
This colored X-ray shows a healthy heart, just behind the lungs and a little to the left.

PETER SELLERS
The comedian and film star, Peter Sellers (1925–80), suffered seven heart attacks within two hours in 1964. But he recovered and went on to star in several more films before he finally died of heart failure 16 years later.

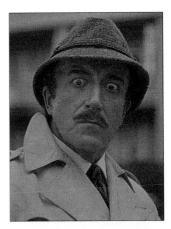

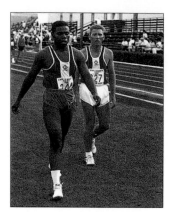

LIFE AFTER A TRANSPLANT
These men, who have had heart transplants, are regular competitors in the British, European, and World Transplant Games. They not only are keen athletes but also participate in transplant support groups, which encourage returning to an active life after surgery.

HEART RELAXATION
Overcoming stress is essential for the health of your heart. Doing relaxation exercises, reading books, and listening to music can all help to combat stress.

angiography. Techniques for countering the effects of damage to the heart are equally innovative; they include bypass operations, angioplasty, valve replacements, pace-makers, and heart transplants and have enabled many heart patients to live reasonably healthy lives. However, treating heart disorders with such methods is expensive and includes the risks of further medical complications. Since most heart disease is caused by damaged arteries as a result of an unhealthy lifestyle, doctors are realizing more and more that changes in lifestyle can both prevent and reverse many cases of heart disease, and patients who acknowledge this are increasingly taking a greater amount of responsibility for their own health.

Before recommending surgery, many specialists now prefer to advise simpler measures, such as changing a patient's diet or developing an exercise program, aimed in both cases at improving the efficiency of the heart and reducing deposits that are clogging the arteries. Now that it is increasingly accepted that the condition of the mind is vital for heart health too, doctors propose treatments that reduce stress—and consequently high blood pressure—and increase cardiovascular efficiency.

MIND OVER MATTER

Statistics are showing that besides lifestyle there is another, and perhaps far greater, determinant of heart disease. Evidence suggests that in addition to being physically unhealthy, many heart patients are leading unhappy lives. People are more vulnerable to premature death from heart disease if they suffer constant stresses in their social and professional environments, if they feel isolated from others, or if they have low or negative self-esteem through feelings of emotional deprivation and psychological inadequacy. Our environments, habits, behavior, and attitudes are all major contributors to the development of heart disease.

As the miss of a beat and a quickening pulse graphically indicate, a disturbance in a person's mind very quickly reverberates in the heart and the entire cardiovascular system. Emotional stress or anxiety can trigger physical stress. How well the cardiovascular system holds up against the extra pressures exerted this way depends on several factors: the level and intensity of the pressures and the individual's genetic tendency, personality and emotional resources, level of physical fitness, and the quality of his or her diet.

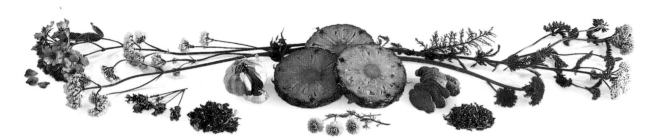

THE HOLISTIC APPROACH

The sensitivity of the heart to personality factors, rather than just issues of medical concern, indicates that cardiovascular problems should be particularly responsive to a broader treatment approach that embraces the psychological along with the physical aspects of health. The conventional medical idea of the body as a system made up of purely mechanical parts has fallen out of favor. The traditional approach to heart treatment, in which blood pressure, cholesterol level, and the structure of the blood vessels are viewed in isolation from personality, is regarded as far too limiting. At least as important are questions about the patient's relationships with family members and work colleagues, the way he or she deals with problems and stressful situations, the way the body is treated, and the success with which the patient can maintain the balance of the physical body, intellectual mind, and emotional spirit.

This is precisely the emphasis of the various natural therapies that holistic medicine is introducing, or in many cases reintroducing, into modern medical practice. These include naturopathy, hydrotherapy, acupuncture, homeopathy, aromatherapy, biofeedback, massage, herbalism, Chinese medicine, and nutrition. Holistic medicine aims to cater to the whole person, beyond the contours of the body and into the patient's psychological and emotional environment. To do this, it dispenses with the conventionally passive role of the patient and encourages a full partnership for health with the doctor or therapist.

The holistic way with heart disease naturally emphasizes prevention first and foremost and seeks to offer treatment that does not require the use of symptom-relieving drugs or interventionist surgery. More important, holism makes many more demands on the patient to develop skills that enable him or her to adapt to the changing circumstances of age, social environment, and pressures of work. To stay physically healthy, we must elaborate methods of coping with the demands made on us to maintain our self-esteem and spiritual well-being.

HEALING HERBS
A number of herbs can play a part in restoring the heart to health. Some can be taken as teas or decoctions, while others, like garlic, onions, and ginger, can be used in cooking. Still other herbs, like lavender, can be added to a bath to aid in relaxation.

BEING SOCIABLE
Many studies have shown that living in social isolation increases the risk of heart disease and slows recovery from heart surgery. Relaxing with your family or friends can help your heart to heal.

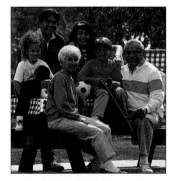

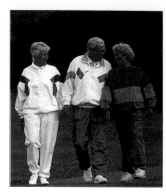

EXERCISE TO HEALTH
Walking briskly for at least 20 minutes three times a week can help lower blood pressure and strengthen your heart. Walking is an essential component of any cardiac rehabilitation program.

FOOT MASSAGE
The first weeks after heart surgery are stressful and uncomfortable. A foot massage is a gentle and effective way to help you relax and recover.

Holism should be seen not as opposed to orthodox healing but rather as complementary to it, to be employed in full cooperation with the advanced methods of technological medicine.

Many heart attacks and strokes need not occur. But lack of information on what can be done to prevent them, passive belief in the capabilities of technological medicine, and a fatalistic resignation to the apparent all-conquering power of heart disease have prevented the general public from appreciating just how much they are responsible for their own health.

The purpose of *A HEALTHY HEART* is to provide you with the knowledge you need in order to make your own decisions on your health and to introduce you to a wider spectrum of care for the heart, in which the roles appropriate to conventional and complementary medicine are given their due place.

After an explanatory chapter on the functioning of the heart and cardiovascular system, *A HEALTHY HEART* is divided into two parts: the first deals with prevention of heart disease, and the second with treatment of it. Chapter 2 describes the many factors that increase the risk of heart disease, such as gender, family history, age, and personality. It also covers lifestyle risks such as smoking, drinking too much, being exposed constantly to high levels of stress, and living a sedentary life; it also provides techniques for stopping smoking and relieving stress. Chapter 3 gives sound advice on how to eat to protect your heart. It provides up-to-date information on the importance of unsaturated fats, antioxidants, fiber, and foods that you should incorporate into your diet if you want to keep your heart healthy. Chapter 4 explains the necessity for regular exercise and tells you how to get moving. It includes illustrated toning and stretching regimens that you can easily follow.

Chapter 5 deals with the diagnosis of heart and circulatory disorders and takes a look at the natural treatment options that are available. Chapter 6 explains these disorders in detail and lists conventional treatments together with alternative therapies that can assist in relieving symptoms. The final chapter discusses recovering after you have had a heart attack or heart surgery, covering such topics as returning to work, resumption of sex, stress management, and ways to control anger—an emotion that often contributes to the development of heart disease.

How much do you really know about heart disease?

Heart disease has received a great deal of media attention over the last three decades, with the result that many people feel they are much more knowledgeable about the subject. But is this really true? The quiz below tests what you know about heart disease. You may be in for one or two surprises.

Q IS IT TRUE THAT DEATHS FROM HEART DISEASE HAVE BEEN RISING STEADILY SINCE THE BEGINNING OF THE CENTURY?

Yes and no. In most Western countries there has been a noticeable rise due to a number of factors, including high-fat diets, an increase in smoking, more sedentary lifestyles, and the effects of stress. In the United States and Canada since the 1960s, however, there has been a decline. It is attributed to a combination of lifestyle changes and advances in medical technology. Conditions that once were invariably fatal are treated far sooner, thus reducing the mortality rate.

Q WHEN I HAD MY BLOOD PRESSURE TAKEN IT WAS 130/85. IS THIS TOO HIGH FOR AN ADULT WHO IS IN REASONABLY GOOD HEALTH?

No, your blood pressure is normal. It is now generally agreed by doctors that a reading that is consistently higher than 140/90 indicates high blood pressure, or hypertension, and warrants therapy because the condition increases the risk of heart attack, heart failure, and stroke. Note, however, that blood pressure in children and the very fit is markedly lower. Blood pressure can rise normally as people grow older but should always be monitored during routine health checks.

Q CAN I LOWER MY CHOLESTEROL LEVEL BY EATING LOW-CHOLESTEROL FOODS?

It may help to eat low-cholesterol foods, but the only way you can greatly reduce your cholesterol is to eat less saturated fat, predominant in animal foods. Monounsaturated and polyunsaturated fats, found in vegetable oils, are preferable because they conserve the "good" (HDL) cholesterol and lower the "bad" (LDL) cholesterol. It also helps to eat more soluble fiber, the kind found in oat and rice brans and many fruits.

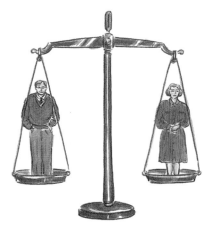

Q IT'S OBVIOUS WHY SMOKING CONTRIBUTES TO LUNG CANCER, BUT WHY SHOULD IT AFFECT THE HEART?

Smoking has a number of negative effects on the heart and other organs, which is why smokers have two to three times the risk of nonsmokers for developing heart disease. The nicotine in cigarettes makes the adrenal glands produce more adrenaline, and this causes an increase in the heart rate and also in blood pressure. The walls of the arteries become constricted, and there is more risk of blood clots and cholesterol buildup. The constriction of the blood vessels in the brain can lead to a stroke.

Q DO MEN AND WOMEN HAVE THE SAME RISK OF HEART DISEASE?

No. Until the menopause women have a lower risk than men because the female hormones, especially estrogen, play a protective role in maintaining levels of "good" cholesterol and lowering levels of "bad" cholesterol. After menopause, when estrogen declines, the levels reverse, and women and men become more equal in risk. In fact, heart disease kills far more women than the dreaded breast cancer.

Q DO YOU ALWAYS KNOW WHEN YOU ARE HAVING A HEART ATTACK?

No. In a few cases, mainly the elderly and diabetics, a heart attack may occur without pain. More typically, though, the pain of a heart attack starts as a mild ache that builds up over half an hour to an hour, becoming more distinct and quite severe. There may be a squeezing feeling in the chest, as well as pain that radiates to the arms and shoulders, sweating, dizziness, nausea, breathlessness, and a feeling of dread. Because 60 percent of heart-attack victims die within the first hour, it is critical that anyone with these symptoms get emergency medical treatment.

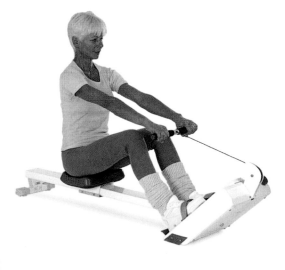

Q WHY IS HIGH-INTENSITY EXERCISE LESS BENEFICIAL FOR THE HEART THAN AEROBIC EXERCISE?

Aerobic exercise, which consists of at least 20 minutes of a vigorous activity like brisk walking, swimming, rowing, and jogging, is best for using oxygen as fuel, for burning fat, and for making the heart pump more efficiently. Anaerobic, or high-intensity, exercise, such as sprinting and weightlifting, which consists of short bursts of activity, does not improve cardiovascular health. In fact, anaerobic exercise may actually put excess strain on an unfit heart.

CHAPTER 1

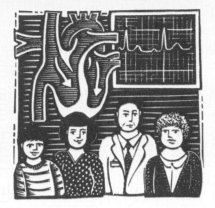

HOW THE HEART WORKS

*From the beginning of life in the womb until
death, the heart works constantly to pump blood
around the body, thus providing the cells with oxygen
and nutrients. An understanding of how the heart and
circulatory system work and what affects their well-
being is essential for maintaining a healthy life.*

THE HEART AND CIRCULATION

At the center of the circulatory system lies the heart, which forces oxygenated blood around the body to every tissue and then receives blood back with carbon dioxide to be expelled.

Figure eight
Blood travels around the body in a figure eight, picking up oxygenated blood from the lungs, sending it out to nourish the body via the arteries, then receiving the blood back through veins and recirculating it to the lungs, where it gives up carbon dioxide and receives more oxygen.

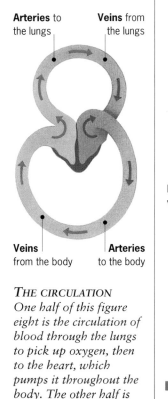

Arteries to the lungs   **Veins** from the lungs

Veins from the body   **Arteries** to the body

THE CIRCULATION
One half of this figure eight is the circulation of blood through the lungs to pick up oxygen, then to the heart, which pumps it throughout the body. The other half is the return of the spent blood to the heart and then the lungs, where it gives up carbon dioxide.

Blood is necessary for the nourishment of every cell in the body. It moves ceaselessly, carrying life-giving oxygen and nutrients from food out to the cells and taking away such waste products as carbon dioxide. The path in which the

THE CIRCULATORY SYSTEM
The heart pumps the blood through the main arteries throughout the body, and it is then returned to the heart via the veins.

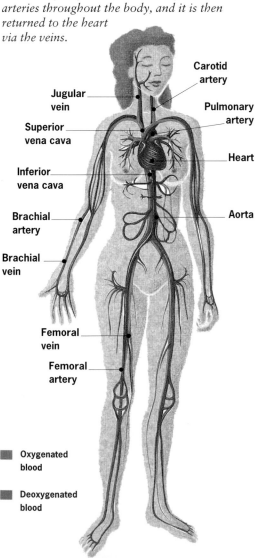

Jugular vein

Carotid artery

Superior vena cava

Pulmonary artery

Inferior vena cava

Heart

Brachial artery

Aorta

Brachial vein

Femoral vein

Femoral artery

■ Oxygenated blood

■ Deoxygenated blood

blood travels around the body is roughly a figure eight, or almost two circles (see illustration, below left). The heart is the pump that keeps this circulating system going.

THE CIRCULATORY SYSTEM
The heart is divided into two parts by a wall called the septum. The left side of the heart helps circulate oxygenated blood, while the right side deals with deoxygenated blood.

The cycle begins in the part known as the "right heart." Here deoxygenated blood (bluish in color) from the body trunk and legs enters the right atrium through a vein called the inferior vena cava, while deoxygenated blood from the head and arms enters the right atrium through another vein, called the superior vena cava. As the walls of the heart contract, blood is pumped down into the right ventricle. When the right ventricle contracts, blood is forced up into the pulmonary artery, which then takes it to the lungs to deposit carbon dioxide and pick up oxygen. (The pulmonary artery is divided into two branches; one leads to the right lung, the other to the left lung.)

The oxygenated blood leaves the lungs and enters the "left heart" through the pulmonary veins; these then take the blood into the left atrium, which contracts, pushing the blood down into the left ventricle. When the thick muscular wall of this ventricle contracts, blood is forced out through the aorta to begin its journey to the rest of the body via the main arteries, such as the femoral arteries in the legs, brachial arteries in the arms, and carotid arteries in the neck.

Once the blood has completed its circuit of the body, it returns to the heart through the superior and inferior venae cavae and enters the right side of the heart, where the

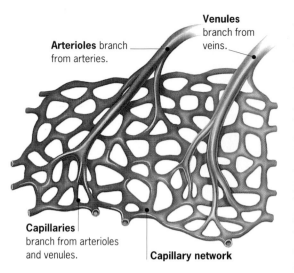

Arterioles branch from arteries.

Venules branch from veins.

Capillaries branch from arterioles and venules.

Capillary network

CAPILLARY NETWORK
Oxygen, nutrients, and waste products pass between the bloodstream and the body tissues via the very thin capillary walls, and blood flows from arteries to veins through the network.

whole process begins again. The heart pumps blood around the body about 70 times a minute every minute of your life. The entire journey of a single blood cell takes just about one minute.

THE BLOOD VESSELS
The circulatory system is made up of an extensive network of blood vessels, which include arteries, arterioles, veins, venules, and capillaries. In total, the length of these vessels is 96,000 km (60,000 miles)!

Arteries
The arteries are thick-walled, muscular tubes through which the blood flows to all parts of the body. As the heart pumps blood through them, they widen, then recoil automatically to push the blood onward, assisting the heart in pushing the blood around the body.

Arteries branch into smaller tubes, or arterioles, which then branch into tiny blood vessels called capillaries. These capillaries link up with venules, which in turn connect with the veins.

Veins
The veins eventually carry blood back to the heart. But by the time the blood reaches the venules and veins, it has run out of pressure. Because veins are not elastic like arteries or able to expand and recoil to force the blood through, most of them have valves that pre-

vent the backflow of blood. It is the movement of muscles surrounding the veins that helps the blood to return to the heart.

Capillaries
Although they keep the tissues supplied with oxygen and nutrients, capillaries are so small that they can hold only a single line of blood cells, and their walls are very thin to allow molecules to pass through them. The pulmonary capillaries allow oxygen from the lung's air sacs, or alveoli, to be absorbed into the blood, which carries the oxygen to the body's cells and exchanges it, via the capillaries, for carbon dioxide. The capillaries link up with the venules, returning carbon dioxide–rich blood through the venous system to the heart, where it is circulated to the lungs again for exhalation of the carbon dioxide it contains.

From the small intestine the blood picks up nutrients, also by way of the capillaries, which have been absorbed from food, exchanging them for waste products that it delivers to the liver or kidneys for excretion.

THE LYMPHATIC SYSTEM
The capillaries exchange fluid with all tissue cells in the process of delivering oxygen and nutrients and taking away carbon dioxide

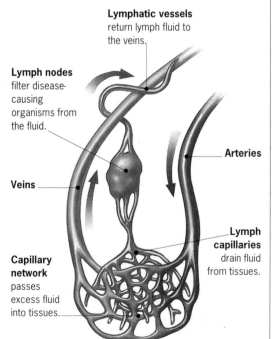

Lymphatic vessels return lymph fluid to the veins.

Lymph nodes filter disease-causing organisms from the fluid.

Arteries

Veins

Lymph capillaries drain fluid from tissues.

Capillary network passes excess fluid into tissues.

LYMPHATIC SYSTEM
The drainage, or lymphatic, system of the body draws off excess fluid from tissue, filters out bacteria and other foreign organisms, and then returns the fluid to the veins.

How the blood carries oxygen
Red blood cells carry hemoglobin, an iron-rich pigment that chemically links with oxygen. When deoxygenated blood passes through the lungs, its hemoglobin picks up the oxygen from the air sacs of the lungs until it has taken up the full complement and has become saturated once more. This oxygen-rich blood is then returned to the heart and pumped out to the tissues. The hemoglobin then gives up its oxygen to cells that are low in oxygen.

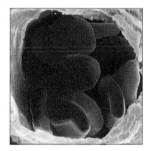

RED BLOOD CELLS
This electron micrograph shows red blood cells traveling through an arteriole. A red blood cell lives for about four months and travels about 15 km (9.3 miles) every day. There are about 5,000 billion red blood cells per liter (quart) of blood.

THE POSITION OF THE HEART

A hollow muscular organ about the size of two fists, the heart sits in the chest, or thoracic, cavity, nestled between the lungs just to the left of the of the chest center. It is protected by the breastbone, or sternum, at the front and the spinal column at the rear.

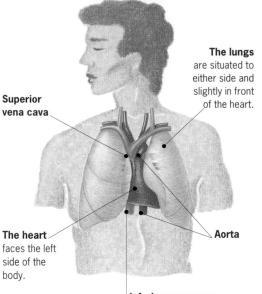

Superior vena cava

The lungs are situated to either side and slightly in front of the heart.

The heart faces the left side of the body.

Aorta

Inferior vena cava

and other waste products. But more fluid passes from capillaries to the tissue cells than returns back to them, so in this exchange the lymphatic drainage system removes excess fluid from the tissues and returns it to the veins via the lymph nodes, where the fluid is filtered for disease-causing organisms.

THE STRUCTURE OF THE HEART

A hollow muscular organ, the heart is made up of four chambers: two atria and two ventricles, with a septum dividing the left side from the right. Blood enters and exits from these chambers by way of valves.

The heart is composed of three layers: the myocardium, which is thick and muscular, and the epicardium and the endocardium, which are thin membranes. The epicardium covers the outer surface of the myocardium, and the endocardium lines the inside of the heart's four chambers, the heart valves, and the muscles that attach to the valves.

How the myocardium works

It is the myocardium, made up of individual muscle cells called myocytes, that actually pumps out the blood. The myocytes direct the entire operation, acting in concert to contract and relax the chambers of the heart in the correct sequence in response to electrical messages that pass between them. Fine threads called filaments contract to shorten the myocytes and thus contract the heart muscle. As the pumping chambers becomes smaller, the blood is squeezed out. When

---

FINDING OUT ABOUT THE HEART

Galen of Pergamon, a Roman who lived in the second century A.D., developed theories about the heart that were accepted for centuries. His belief that blood flowed from one side of the heart to the other remained unchallenged until Andreas Vesalius (1514–64) proved that the heart's septum was solid and thus prevented blood from passing from one side to the other. Vesalius also proposed that blood flowed in a circular, not lateral, route around the body.

William Harvey (1578–1657), an English physician and anatomist, discovered that blood flows from the arteries to the veins and back to

the heart, proving that blood is in constant motion and moves in one direction only.

Harvey based his theories on a mathematical calculation of the heart's output: that is, with each contraction the heart ejects about 59 ml (2 fl oz). Since it beats about 70 times a minute, it would pump about 225 ml (8 fl oz) every hour. Harvey concluded that this was possible only if the blood flowed back to the heart to be pumped out again. Thus he was able to deduce that the heart is a pump and that it keeps the blood moving in a circular direction around the body.

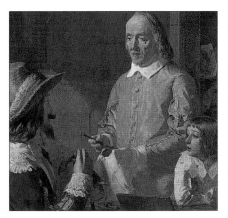

DISCOVERING BLOOD CIRCULATION
William Harvey uses a heart to demonstrate to Charles I in 1628 his theory about circulation of the blood.

THE ANATOMY OF THE HEART

The heart is the hardest-working muscle in the body. From the illustration below you can see that the walls of its ventricles are much thicker than those of the atria because they have to pump blood out to circulate throughout the body. The aorta, the largest blood vessel in the body, carries oxygenated blood; the pulmonary veins carry oxygenated blood, and the pulmonary artery transports deoxygenated blood.

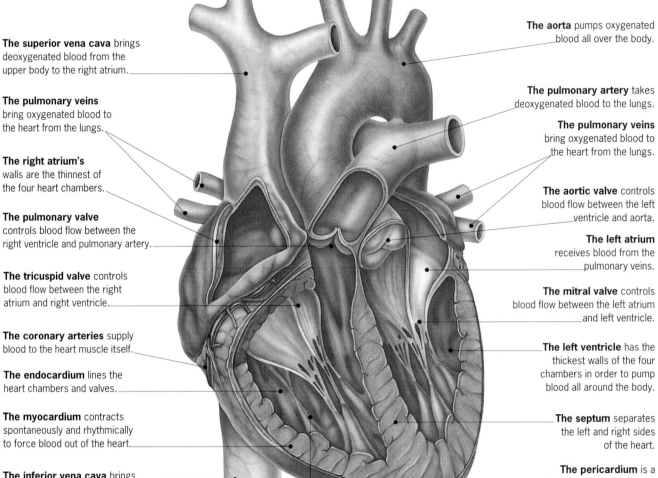

The superior vena cava brings deoxygenated blood from the upper body to the right atrium.

The pulmonary veins bring oxygenated blood to the heart from the lungs.

The right atrium's walls are the thinnest of the four heart chambers.

The pulmonary valve controls blood flow between the right ventricle and pulmonary artery.

The tricuspid valve controls blood flow between the right atrium and right ventricle.

The coronary arteries supply blood to the heart muscle itself.

The endocardium lines the heart chambers and valves.

The myocardium contracts spontaneously and rhythmically to force blood out of the heart.

The inferior vena cava brings deoxygenated blood from the lower body to the right atrium.

The aorta pumps oxygenated blood all over the body.

The pulmonary artery takes deoxygenated blood to the lungs.

The pulmonary veins bring oxygenated blood to the heart from the lungs.

The aortic valve controls blood flow between the left ventricle and aorta.

The left atrium receives blood from the pulmonary veins.

The mitral valve controls blood flow between the left atrium and left ventricle.

The left ventricle has the thickest walls of the four chambers in order to pump blood all around the body.

The septum separates the left and right sides of the heart.

The pericardium is a tough, double-layered membrane surrounding the heart.

The right ventricle pumps deoxygenated blood to the lungs.

the filaments relax, the chambers become larger and fill with blood again. It is this in-and-out process that you feel when you take your pulse or put your hand on your chest.

The pericardium

Covering the entire heart is a bag made of tough fibrous tissue, called the pericardium. It is attached to the large blood vessels emerging from the heart, but not to the heart itself. Unlike the muscles of the heart, the pericardium does not stretch. It is loose-fitting and lined with a moist membrane. The space between the pericardium and the heart contains a tiny amount of lubricating fluid, which allows the heart to expand and contract easily without the danger of irritation from contact with the inner surface of the pericardium.

THE VALVES

The quantity of blood that enters and leaves the heart's left chambers is exactly the same as the amount that passes through the chambers on the right side of the heart. The movement of the blood in and out of the

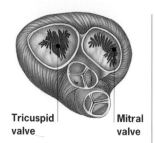

Tricuspid valve　　　**Mitral valve**

BLOOD ENTERS HEART.
This view of the heart from above shows the mitral and tricuspid valves open as blood enters the ventricles from the atria.

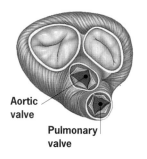

Aortic valve

Pulmonary valve

EXIT OF BLOOD
The aortic valve and pulmonary valve are open here, as blood passes from the left ventricle into the aorta and from the right ventricle into the pulmonary artery.

chambers is controlled by the precise movements of the valves. To keep the blood in the heart flowing in only one direction and at the right rate, the heart has four one-way valves. Each valve has flaps, or cusps, that open to let the blood in and then close to prevent it flowing back the way it came.

The atrioventricular valves guard the openings from the atria into the ventricles. On the right side the tricuspid valve keeps blood from flowing back into the right atrium after it has entered the right ventricle. The mitral valve performs the same function on the left side of the heart. The other two valves—the pulmonary valve between the right ventricle and pulmonary artery and the aortic valve between the left ventricle and aorta—are shaped like half moons. They open and close on cue to keep the blood flowing out of the ventricles to the body at the proper rate.

Heart sounds

In addition to the sound of its beating, the heart makes a number of other noises that are audible with amplification. The stethoscope is the most commonly used amplifying device. Abnormal heart sounds, such as clicks, snaps, murmurs, or whooshes, can indicate disorders of the heart, and your doctor may investigate them further.

By listening at four different places on the chest, your doctor can hear sounds made by the four heart valves opening and closing in rhythm. In a normal heart there are two

sounds, known as lubb and dupp. One of the sounds is caused by the slamming shut of the tricuspid and mitral valves. The other occurs when the aortic and pulmonary valves shut. In young adults and children, the second sound may be split because the two valves do not close at exactly the same time, but this is normal and not dangerous.

A rushing sound, or heart murmur, is abnormal and is caused by turbulent blood flow. This particular noise may suggest that there are problems with one of the heart valves. Heart murmurs are more common in children but are also found in adults. They sometimes occur in newborn babies and usually disappear within a few days, although they can indicate a congenital heart defect (see page 106).

HOW THE HEART BEATS

The heart beats an average of 70 times per minute. The timing of the heartbeat is controlled by the sinoatrial (sinus) node, a group of cells located in the upper part of the right atrium. This is the heart's natural pacemaker. In a healthy heart the sinoatrial node directs the heart's conduction system (see opposite) and maintains a regular rhythm. Its cells send out electrical impulses that make the heart muscle contract, and their rate of discharge is modulated by nerve impulses from the brain.

Electric current is both initiated and controlled from the sinoatrial node. The current travels first to the atria and then to the atrioventricular node and is passed on from there to the ventricles. The group of nerves that make up the electrical network of the ventricles is called the His-Purkinje system, and its job is to direct the current through the cells in both ventricles.

To make sure that the atria contract before the ventricles, the atrioventricular node slows down the current. The time required for the electrical impulse occurring in the sinoatrial node to reach the myocardial cells averages about one-quarter of a second in a heart beating 70 times a minute.

The rate set by the sinoatrial node changes according to the demands of the body. It can increase the heartbeat from an average of about 70 beats per minute when resting to about 180 beats per minute during strenuous exercise, and it slows down the heart while you rest or sleep. Other impulses and hormonal activity can also affect the pace

LISTENING TO THE HEART

A doctor will place a stethoscope at four different positions on your chest, which correspond to the four valves.

A diagnosis is made, depending on which noises are heard. Further tests may be needed to confirm the diagnosis.

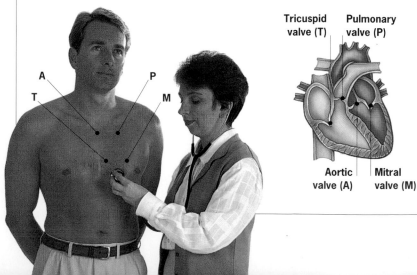

A　　P

T　　M

Tricuspid valve (T)　　**Pulmonary valve (P)**

Aortic valve (A)　　**Mitral valve (M)**

that the sinoatrial node sets. Factors such as smoking, consumption of alcohol or caffeine, as well as some prescription drugs, speed the heartbeat by affecting the sympathetic nervous system (see below) and hormones such as adrenaline.

THE PULSE

Your heart beats about 100,000 times a day throughout your life. Each beat can be felt as a pulse at points on the body where arteries lie close to the surface of the skin.

The flow of blood in the arteries increases as a new volume of blood is pumped into them with each heartbeat. The arterial walls expand when blood enters them and then recoil when it empties into the capillaries, thus creating a pulse. The pulse can be felt most easily over a bone or other firm spot where an artery lies, such as in the wrist and neck. The pulse can also be felt at points just in front of the ear, on the outer side of the eye, and on the upper surface of the foot.

CARDIAC OUTPUT

Even though it beats constantly, the heart does not pump all the blood from the ventricles at any one time. The proportion that leaves the heart when it contracts is called the ejection fraction and consists of about half the blood in the ventricle. The ejection fraction in a healthy body increases by about 5 to 10 percent when there are increased demands for oxygen made on the heart, such as during exercise or times of stress.

The stroke volume is the amount of blood that is pumped into the aorta by the left ventricle in one contraction. The cardiac output is the total volume of blood pumped by the heart in one minute. It is determined by the heart rate (the number of heartbeats per minute) and the stroke volume.

When you exercise, not only does the heart pump more often but it also contracts more forcefully, and the muscle stretches so that more blood is pumped with each beat and the overall cardiac output increases.

The coronary arteries, which are the fuel lines of the heart, stem from the aorta and provide blood to the heart muscle itself. These arteries form a crown that encircles the top of the heart and runs along its surface. They then divide into increasingly smaller branches that penetrate the heart muscle. Finally the branches become capillaries, in which the blood's oxygen and nutrients are exchanged for waste products. Blood flow through the coronary arteries averages 200 ml (7 fl oz) per minute. The heart uses 4 to 5 percent of the blood it pumps.

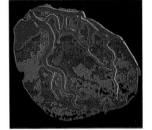

HEART IMAGE
This scan shows mostly healthy coronary arteries, but one artery, in the top right-hand corner, shows an abnormal narrowing (stenosis). When fatty deposits build up in these arteries because of unhealthy eating habits, they become blocked.

THE CONDUCTION SYSTEM

Nerve impulses pass from the sinoatrial node to the atria, then to the atrioventricular node and on to the ventricles. The brain, in response to the nervous system, regulates the sinoatrial node. The sympathetic nervous system, which prepares the body for action, speeds up the heart in response to stress or exercise; the parasympathetic nervous system, which regulates processes such as digestion, slows it down.

The sinoatrial node controls the heart rate and rhythm of contractions.

The atrioventricular node passes electrical signals from the atria to the ventricles.

The His-Purkinje system of nerves sends signals to the ventricle cells.

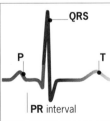

AN ECG READING represents electrical pathways in the heart. The P wave shows the impulse traveling through the atrium; the PR interval, as it passes through the atrioventricular node; the QRS complex, as it travels through the ventricles; and the T wave, as the heart relaxes before the next beat (see page 91).

BLOOD PRESSURE

The heart pushes blood through the circulatory system with great force. Without this pressure, the blood would not be able to reach every part of the body.

Blood pressure measurements

Blood pressure is recorded in millimeters of mercury (mm Hg) because the earliest devices for measuring blood pressure used a column of mercury calibrated against a millimeter scale.

The heart's action of pumping blood is called a systole. With each heartbeat blood surges through the arteries and arterioles, and pressure is at its highest; this is systolic pressure. It is then followed by a very short pause, called a diastole, which occurs between heartbeats when the pressure is at its lowest. This low period is referred to as diastolic pressure.

The heart muscle rests during diastole so that the heart cavities can dilate and fill with blood before the heart contracts once again and forces blood into the arteries. At a heart rate of 70 beats per minute, the diastole, or rest period, is normally about three-fifths of a second.

The arteries, which carry blood away from the heart, are normally resilient and elastic and able to withstand the varying flow of blood as the heart pumps. The two pressures audible in the heartbeat, the diastolic (resting phase) and systolic (pumping phase), remain within normal limits when the blood flow from the heart neither meets nor creates too much resistance in the arteries. However, if artery walls become inflexible, any additional fluid will cause a rise in pressure because more blood is forced through a confined space. This can result in serious health problems.

High blood pressure

Blood pressure is naturally elevated during exercise or exertion because the heart has to pump more blood to supply muscles, but this effect is only temporary. When arteries narrow or become rigid because of disease or aging, however, the walls cannot expand to relieve pressure, so blood pressure rises and remains elevated over time. This condition is known as high blood pressure, or hypertension. Unless it is treated, high blood pressure itself further damages the artery walls, making them even less elastic, which drives the blood pressure up even more.

High blood pressure is symptomless in the majority of cases but may sometimes cause headaches, giddiness, visual disturbances, and shortness of breath.

Low blood pressure

Blood pressure that is lower than normal (see opposite) is known as hypotension and usually causes no problems, apart from occasional lightheadedness or fainting. Very fit people often have low blood pressure, as do young women. Blood pressure that is dangerously low (a systolic pressure less than 60 mm Hg) is usually associated with shock or serious bleeding.

WHAT INFLUENCES BLOOD PRESSURE

Blood pressure rises when the heart pumps blood into the arteries at an increased rate (as during exercise) or if arteries are constricted and thus resist blood flow from the heart.

Healthy diastolic pressure is no more than 90.

Diastolic pressure over 95 indicates hypertension.

Systolic pressure less than 60 can be dangerous.

Elastic arteries

Narrowed arteries

Widened arteries

Healthy arteries are elastic and expand and contract easily, keeping blood pressure normal.

Narrowed arteries, which result from disease or aging, cause blood pressure to rise.

Arteries widen more than usual when a person bleeds heavily or is in shock and cause blood pressure to drop.

MAINTAINING A NORMAL BLOOD PRESSURE

Keeping your blood pressure at a healthy level is of paramount importance to avoid damaging the artery walls and raising the risk of heart disease and stroke. Medical professionals and other scientists agree that maintaining a healthy diet, exercising regularly, and avoiding excessive stress can all contribute to keeping blood pressure low or help to lower it if it has become too high.

People who are at risk for high blood pressure should have regular checkups. Risk factors include obesity, taking contraceptive pills, smoking, excessive alcohol intake, a family history of the disease, pregnancy, and constant stress. To monitor the impact of lifestyle changes, some people have blood pressure machines at home (see page 96), but this is not usually necessary.

If your blood pressure is high, your doctor will advise changes in diet and lifestyle and may prescribe medication. Foods especially good for the heart are vegetables, fruits, and fish. Fats should be limited, particularly the saturated fats in dairy products and red meat. Moderation in all things, particularly in consumption of salt and alcohol, is also important. Smoking, too, must be avoided.

MEASURING BLOOD PRESSURE

Attempts have been made to measure blood pressure since the 19th century. In 1863 Etienne-Jules Marey of Paris introduced the first practical instrument to measure the way the blood pulsed and the amount of pressure in the arteries. The instrument, which was called a sphygmograph, contained an arrangement of screws and levers for altering tensions on the arm. Other scientists improved on Marey's design.

Blood pressure is now measured with an instrument called a sphygmomanometer, which is a refinement on Marey's early efforts. It measures pressure in the brachial artery of the upper arm. A cuff attached by rubber tubes to a squeezeable bulb and a column of mercury (some devices have a round dial instead) is wrapped around the arm and inflated until no blood can flow through the artery. Pressure in the cuff is then slowly released, and the doctor listens with a stethoscope placed over the artery below the cuff. As blood starts to flow, it creates a thumping noise and the pressure in the cuff at this time is recorded as the systolic pressure. As pressure in the cuff falls farther, the sound suddenly becomes muffled and then disappears as blood flow is no longer obstructed. This is the time when a reading of the diastolic pressure is taken.

Normal adult pressure readings register below 140 systolic pressure and 90 diastolic pressure, recorded as 140/90. Healthy, young people, young women in particular, usually have lower readings. Anything consistently higher than 140/90 is defined as hypertension and requires lifestyle changes and/or medical treatment. To make a firm diagnosis, blood pressure should be measured several times over a number of weeks unless the initial reading is dangerously high (160/110). Blood pressure can be measured at home with an instrument that has an internal listening device and a digital readout.

BLOOD PRESSURE READING
A health practitioner will place a cuff on your arm and listen to the blood pressure changes. A reading is more accurate if you are calm and relaxed while your blood pressure is being measured.

Blood pressure
When blood pressure is measured, figures are read for both systolic and diastolic pressure.

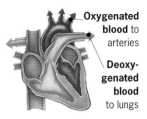
Oxygenated blood to arteries
Deoxygenated blood to lungs

SYSTOLE
When ventricles contract and force blood into the arteries, arterial blood pressure is at its highest; this is called systolic pressure.

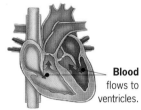
Blood flows to ventricles.

DIASTOLE
Blood flows into the ventricles from the atria as the heart relaxes between beats. Arterial blood pressure is then at its lowest and is called diastolic pressure.

Cuff is inflated on arm.
Pressure is read off the gauge.

A HEART FOR ALL SEASONS

Throughout life your heart must adjust to biological, psychological, and environmental changes. It starts out beating rapidly in childhood, then slows down in adulthood.

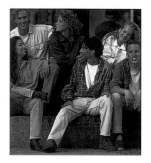

THE HEART IN ADOLESCENCE
Prior to adolescence boys and girls have similar heart rates. During adolescence, however, girls have a higher resting heart rate.

BLOOD PRESSURE AND ADOLESCENCE
Systolic blood pressure in girls rises rapidly until menstruation begins and then levels off. Systolic pressure also rises steadily in boys before puberty, but the change is not as dramatic as for girls. Diastolic pressure does not fluctuate much for either boys or girls.

The heart of a fetus begins to beat approximately 20 days after conception. It can first be heard at about eight weeks, and the heart rate at this stage is between 140 and 150 beats per minute (bpm)—approximately twice that of the mother's resting heart rate.

HEART DEVELOPMENT
The fetal circulatory system, which begins to develop in the second week, is well established at eight weeks, and the heart has already developed into a four-chamber pump, strong enough to pump the embryo's blood around its network of blood vessels.

It is during the first eight weeks of life that the fetal heart is most vulnerable to outside influences, such as illness in the mother or X-rays. However, fewer than 1 percent of babies have heart defects at birth (see Congenital Heart Disorders, page 106). These may be detected during routine ultrasound, or may be noticed only when a newborn is being examined by a doctor.

By the end of the 12th week of gestation, the fetus has started to produce its own blood cells in preparation for taking over an independent system of nourishment. By the 28th week, the baby has taken over full responsibility for the production of its own red blood cells. At birth a baby's heart and circulatory system are fully functional and continue to grow with the rest of the body throughout childhood until adolescence.

Adolescence
At the onset of adolescence, there are various noticeable changes in blood pressure, heart rate, and other physiological functions. For both boys and girls, systolic blood pressure rises steadily until puberty but then levels off. Diastolic pressure does not change much. The rise in systolic pressure occurs earlier in girls than in boys and the changes are more dramatic, but systolic pressure is ultimately higher in men. As blood pressure increases throughout the growing years, there is a corresponding decrease in the heart rate. During adolescence girls have a heart rate that is 10 percent higher than that of boys at the same age. In adulthood women continue to have a higher resting heart rate than men.

Adulthood
Women tend to have smaller hearts and narrower coronary arteries than men. Some doctors believe that this size difference makes

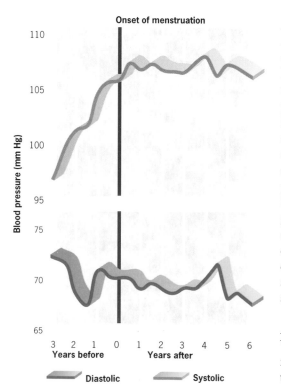

Onset of menstruation

Blood pressure (mm Hg)

110
105
100
95
75
70
65

3 2 1 0 1 2 3 4 5 6
Years before — **Years after**

━━ **Diastolic**   ━━ **Systolic**

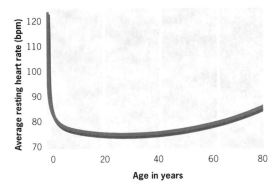

HEART RATE AND AGE
A newborn baby has a heart rate of about 120 bpm. This decreases sharply until the thirties, when it begins to rise again more gradually.

women more susceptible to the effects of atherosclerosis (hardening of the arteries). There is also some evidence that suggests women's coronary arteries contract more strongly than men's as a response to stress.

If size puts women at a disadvantage, the female hormone estrogen puts them at a distinct advantage. It seems to protect women against cardiac disease until its production drops dramatically after menopause. This is the reason that women do not have as many heart attacks as men until past age 65, when differences between the sexes are no longer a factor in heart disease (see page 29).

THE DEMANDS OF PREGNANCY

The body has a remarkable ability to adapt to change. At no time is this more apparent than during pregnancy. The heart and circulatory systems adjust themselves to make nourishment of the fetus possible throughout the nine months of pregnancy.

During this period the mother's blood volume increases to 30 to 40 percent above nonpregnant levels and can rise to 50 percent above normal by the 32nd week of gestation. A pregnant woman carries 1.2 to 1.7 liters (2 to 3 pints) more body fluid than she usually does. At about 34 weeks of gestation, the blood volume reaches its maximum limit and remains at that level throughout the rest of pregnancy.

The extra volume of blood creates more work for the heart, which must pump it to the developing fetus as well as the mother's body. The heart beats faster, pumping out more blood with each contraction (cardiac output) in order to handle this extra load. An expectant mother's pulse rate when measured at rest is 10 to 15 beats higher than that of a woman who is not pregnant.

Blood pressure in the arteries is affected by the woman's position. It is highest when she is seated or standing and lowest when she is lying on her back. Blood pressure is usually lowest during the second, or middle, trimester of pregnancy and rises from that time on. Pressure in the veins, however, is not affected by pregnancy and remains unchanged. Despite this circumstance, a pregnant woman is prone to varicose veins because her uterus may impair the return flow of blood from the legs, thus causing the veins to swell. Because high blood pressure can give rise to dangerous complications during pregnancy, blood pressure should be checked regularly (see page 41).

AGING AND THE HEART

Aging can have two main effects on the heart: an increase in rate (cardiac output) and a reduction in the amount of blood pumped with each beat (stroke volume, see page 21).

PREGNANCY AND CIRCULATION
A mother's blood supplies oxygen and nutrients to her baby via the placenta. Both baby and placenta require 25 percent of the mother's cardiac output.

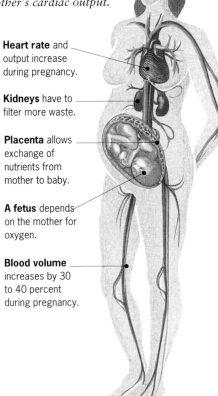

Heart rate and output increase during pregnancy.

Kidneys have to filter more waste.

Placenta allows exchange of nutrients from mother to baby.

A fetus depends on the mother for oxygen.

Blood volume increases by 30 to 40 percent during pregnancy.

Is treatment necessary?

Although blood pressure naturally rises with age in many people, studies show that it is worth treating even mild hypertension because keeping blood pressure levels down markedly reduces the risk of stroke and heart disease in people over age 65. Treatment does not necessarily mean medication. There are several other measures that can be tried first, including losing weight; giving up smoking; cutting down on fat, salt, and alcohol; learning to relax; and exercising regularly.

Atherosclerosis

As arteries grow older and more rigid, fats are more likely to attach to them and form plaques.

Fats in blood

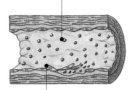

Cells lining artery

DAMAGED WALLS
When the cells lining artery walls become damaged, fats (including cholesterol) build up.

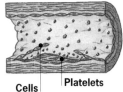

Cells lining artery | **Platelets**

PLAQUES FORM
White blood cells and platelets get stuck on the fatty deposits and the artery narrows.

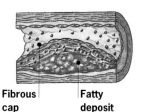

Fibrous cap | **Fatty deposit**

FURTHER BLOCKAGE
A fibrous cap forms over the fatty deposit. Blood clots may form in the narrowed artery.

The heart muscle becomes progressively weaker and therefore less efficient. At the same time the aorta (main artery of the body) becomes less elastic. These aging processes of the heart start at age 20, after which the heart loses nearly 1 percent of muscle strength every year. Three other changes that occur with age include thickening of the heart valves, increased blood pressure, and atherosclerosis (fatty deposits in the arteries); these are not inevitable but are related to lifestyle.

Such changes may sound depressing, but the decreasing efficiency of the heart is offset by a drop in the metabolic rate and less intense demands by the body to respond to activity. However, the heart's ability to cope with stress is impeded because arteries are less elastic and do not respond as well to fluctuating blood pressure (see page 22).

Aging arteries

High-fat diets, as well as several other unhealthy habits that are common in the Western world, mean that even children and teenagers may have fatty streaks in their arteries. After the age of 20, fibrous plaque is more likely to develop, and between 30 and 45, the plaques may become calcified, especially when a person is inactive and has a poor diet. After this time heart problems may develop, depending on other risk factors, such as smoking, amount of exercise, and family history.

Blood pressure and age

Healthy blood pressure levels are relative to age. In Western countries blood pressure tends to rise until people are in their seventies, and then levels off. A blood pressure reading of 160/100 would be considered hypertension in a young person but would be more usual in a person over 80 because of the natural aging of the arteries. It should, however, be reduced if possible.

Although fewer than 3 percent of children suffer from high blood pressure, if the condition begins in childhood, it may go undetected for many years. This could then lead to serious problems in later life. All cases of elevated blood pressure in youngsters under 10 should be investigated. Often there is a specific and treatable cause. A child under 6 years of age should have a blood pressure of about 110/75; between 6 and 10 years a normal reading is 120/80.

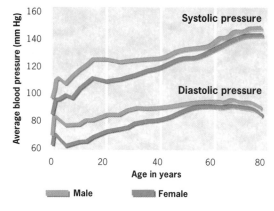

CHANGING BLOOD PRESSURE
Blood pressure tends to rise with age in Western populations, in large part because of high-fat diets, too little exercise, too much stress, and unhealthy habits like smoking.

In some populations, such as the Fijians, the Amazon Indians, the Bushmen in the Kalahari, and the highlanders in New Guinea, there has been no association between age and rising blood pressure.

Lifestyle factors—such as diet, smoking, alcohol, exercise, and stress—play a large part in determining the effect of aging on blood pressure levels. You can keep your own blood pressure relatively healthy by following the lifestyle recommendations in the next chapter.

HEART DISEASE AND AGE

Heart disease is most common among the middle-aged and elderly. Typical changes that occur in the heart with age, like the arteries becoming blocked with fat or damaged by high blood pressure, may contribute to coronary heart disease, the most common heart problem in older patients.

There are, however, some forms of heart disease that occur in babies (see Congenital Heart Disorders, page 106), and sometimes teenagers and young adults are affected, most commonly by rheumatic heart disease, which is caused by a throat infection (see page 117). Heart diseases are covered in more detail in chapter 6.

Although the heart and circulatory systems inevitably show signs of wear and tear as they age, you can keep yours in reasonably good health by controlling weight, blood pressure, and cholesterol levels; getting regular exercise; giving up smoking; and cutting down on alcohol. Managing stress is also essential for preventing damage to the heart.

CHAPTER 2

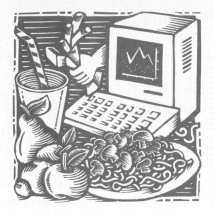

LIFESTYLE AND A HEALTHY HEART

Keeping your heart well is one of the many good reasons for maintaining a healthy lifestyle. Diet, exercise, and habits all play a part in the heart's health. Factors such as gender, personality type, and a family history of heart disease cannot be changed, but a healthy lifestyle can go a long way toward controlling these risks.

WHO IS AT RISK FOR HEART DISEASE?

Many deaths from heart disease can be prevented if people modify the way they live. However, there are some factors for the problem that are impossible to change.

The contraceptive pill
Early oral contraceptive pills increased the risk of heart disease by raising blood pressure, blood cholesterol levels, and the blood's tendency to clot. Although present versions contain lower doses of hormones, women who are on the pill should have their blood pressure taken when getting a new supply. And if they smoke, they should quit, because smoking can also lead to high blood pressure.

There are several risk factors that increase the likelihood of suffering a heart attack. Two ground-breaking research projects—the Ancel Keys Seven Countries Study (Finland, Greece, Italy, Japan, Netherlands, United States, and the former Yugoslavia) and the Framingham Study (suburb of Boston)—provided much information on reducing risk factors. The Seven Countries Study (1957–62) of 12,000 men aged 40 to 59 years showed the importance of blood cholesterol as a risk factor for heart disease. The main findings of the Framingham Study (ongoing since 1948) of 5,000 men and women over 40 years old confirmed the contributions of smoking, cholesterol, and high blood pressure. All of these risk factors can be changed and are therefore known as lifestyle or acquired risk factors. Physical inactivity is another important acquired risk factor.

Those who stop smoking, restrict their intake of dietary fat, exercise regularly, and follow advice on reducing high blood pressure will reduce their coronary risks. The benefits of following these guidelines are greatest for people who are at a particularly high risk and for younger people.

Unfortunately, there are major risk factors for heart disease that cannot be changed. These include being male, having a family history of the disease, having diabetes, being a member of certain ethnic groups, personality type, and increasing age.

HEART DISEASE LEAGUE

Among the industrial nations Japan has the lowest risk of death from heart disease, followed closely by China. This chart, which shows how some other countries compared to Japan between 1985 and 1987, resulted from a major international World Health Organization study that looked at coronary heart disease death rates per 100,000 population.

Among both men and women, the death rates from heart disease were the highest in Scotland and Northern Ireland, while the lowest rates were seen in France and Italy. Differences among the countries are attributed mainly to dietary factors, with the Mediterranean diet ranking high as a preventive (see page 56).

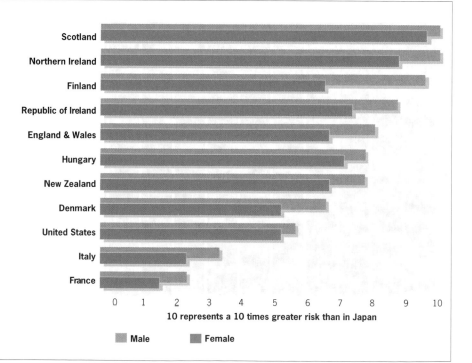

10 represents a 10 times greater risk than in Japan

Male ▪ Female

GENDER

Coronary heart disease is often thought of as a man's problem. It is true that between ages 35 and 44, a man is five or six times more likely to die from this condition than a woman. But in countries where heart disease is a major problem, it kills more women than any other disease. Every year in North America at least five times as many women die from heart attacks as from breast cancer.

Women and coronary heart disease

Women with heart disease are more likely to die from it than men. This is partly because they are older when they develop heart problems and partly because heart disease is perceived as a man's problem. The result is that symptoms of this condition in women are generally taken less seriously by doctors, who may assume that a complaint of chest pain is psychosomatic (about one-third of women in the United States have heart attacks that are not identified). Studies have shown that women with symptoms of heart disease are less likely to be referred to a hospital for diagnosis and treatment and are less often treated with surgery than men with the same condition.

Menopause

A woman's risk of dying from heart disease increases dramatically after she stops menstruating. This is because production of female hormones, particularly estrogen, which offer some protection against heart disease, drops significantly after menopause. After the age of 65, the risk of dying from heart disease is almost the same for women as it is for men.

Although the mechanism is not understood, estrogen in premenopausal women helps maintain high levels of high-density lipoproteins (HDLs), the "good" cholesterol, and low levels of low-density lipopro-

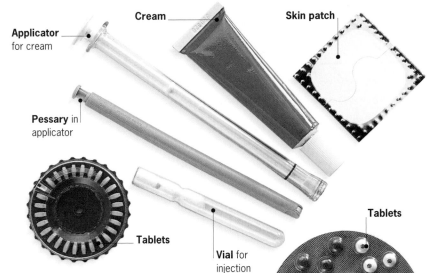

Applicator for cream

Cream

Skin patch

Pessary in applicator

Tablets

Vial for injection

Tablets

HRT
HRT can be administered as tablets, a skin cream, a skin patch, an implant, or a vaginal cream or pessary.

teins (LDLs), the "bad" cholesterol, thus reducing the risk of heart disease (see page 38). After menopause this situation reverses; HDL levels decrease and LDL levels rise, thus increasing the risk of heart problems.

However, studies have shown that post-menopausal women who receive hormone replacement therapy (HRT) in the estrogen-only form can reduce their coronary risk by up to 50 percent. Hormone replacement therapy reduces total blood cholesterol and increases HDL cholesterol. Unfortunately, HRT can elevate triglycerides (see page 53) as well, high levels of which are also bad for the heart and may be related to an increased risk of uterine cancer.

Another form of HRT, which is a combination of estrogen plus progestogen (a synthetic form of progesterone), may offer protection from the triglyceride and cancer effects but has other side effects. Newer forms of HRT are still being researched to maximize benefits and minimize side effects.

FAMILY HISTORY

Coronary heart disease sometimes runs in families. Studies have suggested that if your father or brother has a heart attack before the age of 50 or if your mother or sister has a coronary before 55, your risk of having a heart attack may be doubled or possibly even quadrupled. Scientists do not believe there is a specific genetic factor responsible for familial clusterings of coronary heart disease. Rather, it is probable that there are combinations of certain genes that affect the risk factors for the disease, such as high

continued on page 32

Why take HRT?

About 20 percent of women experience unpleasant symptoms after menopause from the sudden reduction in estrogen levels. These include hot flashes, night sweats, loss of vaginal moisture, decreased libido, fatigue, depression, and irritability. The drop in estrogen levels can also contribute to the onset of osteoporosis (bone-thinning disease) and atherosclerosis. Individual symptoms may be treated, or your doctor may advise you to take HRT. However, women who have had cancer of the breast or uterus will not usually be given HRT because it may lead to a recurrence.

DID YOU KNOW?
Race plays an important part in determining the risk for coronary heart disease. For reasons that are unclear, the percentage of African Americans with hypertension is 50 percent greater than that of whites or Asians, and they are more likely to suffer congestive heart failure.

A Postmenopausal Woman

After menopause, when estrogen levels fall, a woman's risk of heart disease increases because estrogen protects the heart. It is therefore vital that her blood pressure and blood cholesterol levels be monitored regularly. Women who have several risk factors for heart disease should consider hormone replacement therapy (HRT) to reduce the risk.

At 58 Lesley feels that she leads a fairly normal life with husband Ronald, a married daughter Jenny, and three grandchildren. She has smoked throughout her married life, but never more than 15 cigarettes a day, and would be the first to admit she is overweight, though not excessively so; anyway, Ronald says he likes her like that. She often tries out the latest diet but soon lapses, snacking on cookies, chips, and candy, especially when busy.

Her job as a consultant for a computer company involves entertaining, so she often drinks slightly more than is wise, but aside from high blood pressure, for which she is taking medication, her health is reasonably good.

Lesley went through menopause in her early fifties, but unlike her friends, she was fortunate not to suffer serious symptoms, such as depression, mood swings, night sweats, or hot flashes.

Though she has never been very interested in sports or fitness routines, Lesley feels she is still very active. She enjoys gardening—when she has time—and is often called on to look after her energetic grandchildren.

Her daughter and son-in-law both have very busy careers and enjoy a full social life, so she also helps out with some of their domestic chores, but she is beginning to find this activity too much of a strain.

She is thinking of retiring, but because of recent redundancies at her husband's firm, she is starting to worry about the future and how they will manage financially. Recently she has been suffering chest pains and occasional panic attacks.

Both her parents died of heart disease in their sixties, and Lesley is frightened that she might too.

FAMILY
Even after they are grown up, children often remain dependent on parents and forget that they may also need support.

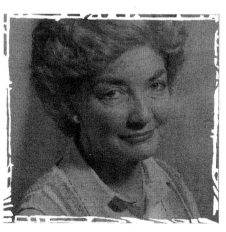

DIET
When you are busy with work and household chores, it's easy to neglect your diet in favor of high-fat snacks. Too much fat increases the risk of heart disease.

EMOTIONAL HEALTH
The link between mental stress and heart disease is well known. Yet people invariably wait until serious symptoms appear before acting.

MEDICATION
Women often do not realize that the risk of heart disease increases after menopause but that hormone replacement therapy can help reduce this risk.

EXERCISE
Many people associate exercise only with strenuous activities, such as aerobics or jogging. As they age, people often feel such pursuits are beyond them and so become increasingly inactive.

WHAT SHOULD LESLEY DO?

Lesley should visit her doctor immediately to discuss her health and lifestyle and to talk over any family problems that are worrying her.

The doctor will want to carry out a thorough physical examination, including exercise stress tests to check Lesley's heart and lungs. She will measure her blood pressure and take blood samples to test cholesterol levels and also to discover whether Lesley has already suffered heart damage (painless heart attacks are more common in women than men).

In view of Lesley's family history of heart disease, she should discuss with the doctor whether hormone replacement therapy is appropriate for her. Estrogen therapy has been shown to reduce the risk of coronary heart disease in postmenopausal women by up to 50 percent, but it may have risks.

Lesley must also make major lifestyle changes. Having a somewhat unhealthy diet, relatively high blood pressure, and a smoking habit; being overweight; and consuming alcohol above recommended levels all combine to increase the likelihood of heart disease. The stress in her life is an added risk factor. Constantly high stress levels increase the risk of heart problems and may cause angina, although in Lesley's case the chest pain was actually caused by her panic attacks.

Action Plan

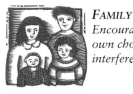
FAMILY
Encourage family members to take responsibility for their own chores and arrangements. Help only when it does not interfere with exercise program and personal commitments.

EMOTIONAL HEALTH
Identify sources of stress and find ways to manage them, such as exercising regularly and doing deep breathing exercises. Spend more time on own activities.

DIET
Improve diet by eating low-fat snacks like fruit and raw vegetables. Do not buy any more sweet and fatty foods and ask friends to help by not offering anything tempting.

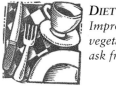
EXERCISE
Walk for at least 20 minutes three times a week and go to a local swimming pool with Ronald on weekends. Walk instead of catching a bus when there is time. Use stairs, not elevators.

MEDICATION
Visit doctor after the first cycle of HRT and again at three months for a checkup to make sure that the medication is the right combination. Tell doctor about any severe side effects.

HOW THINGS TURNED OUT FOR LESLEY

Lesley was started on a course of hormone replacement therapy with skin patches. The doctor prescribed a combination of estrogen and progestogen, as this minimized the possible danger of cancer of the uterus that might arise with estrogen therapy alone.

Lesley attended a woman's health clinic for a diet and exercise program designed to reduce her weight and cholesterol levels and strengthen her heart. The diet involved reduced levels of fat and increased amounts of vegetables, fruits, and complex carbohydrates.

She began regular sessions of walking and swimming, building up to 20-minute sessions three times a week, to give her heart a boost and lower her stress levels.

Lesley reduced her alcohol intake, and with hypnotherapy she gave up smoking.

At Lesley's request, her daughter and son-in-law stopped calling on her to help out as often as before. Lesley and Ronald also looked at their finances and realized that their pension scheme and savings would enable them to live a reasonably comfortable life if she retired. Ronald also started to exercise and cut down on smoking.

Lesley's panic attacks stopped after two months, and her chest pain disappeared. Together with Ronald she was able to spend more time doing things she enjoyed.

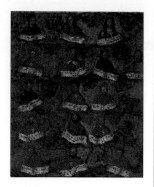

FAMILY TREE
Inherited medical conditions like familial hyperlipoproteinemia can increase the risk of a heart attack. It is important to be aware of your family history in order to inform your doctor of any possible risk factors. You may wish to construct your own family tree and find out what conditions run in your family.

blood cholesterol or high blood pressure. Environmental influences can also play a role; for instance, poor eating habits may be passed on from parent to child.

Hyperlipoproteinemia

Hyperlipoproteinemia—also called hyperlipidemia or hyperlipemia—refers to a range of disorders in which there is too much fat in the blood. It may result from excess fat in the diet or be associated with a disease like diabetes or hypothyroidism, but sometimes it is caused by an inherited chemical defect.

Familial hypercholesterolemia (FH) is the most serious form of hyperlipoproteinemia, and the gene is inherited in a dominant manner; if one parent has the FH gene, the chances are that half of the children in the family will inherit it. All children of a diagnosed individual should be tested for the disease because it requires special care, beginning in early childhood. The condition can be detected at birth if a sample of umbilical cord blood is taken and cholesterol levels are measured. Individuals with FH are at an increased risk of early death from coronary heart disease; it is possible for FH sufferers as young as 20 to have heart problems.

The disease is usually treated by a combination of diet and drug therapy. In most cases, cholesterol-lowering drugs are essential, but many FH sufferers can decrease their risk of coronary heart disease significantly by following a lifelong diet that is low in cholesterol and saturated fat. Also, they should never smoke or take the contraceptive pill without medical advice.

DIABETES

Diabetes mellitus is a metabolic condition in which the body either does not produce or does not fully utilize insulin. There are two kinds. Insulin-dependent, or Type I, diabetes occurs in children and young adults and is controlled with daily injections of insulin. Noninsulin-dependent, also called Type II or adult-onset, diabetes is most common among overweight older people, but it can occur in persons of normal weight. It is largely controlled by exercise and diet; however, medication is sometimes necessary. People with diabetes are at an increased risk of kidney disease, blindness, and nerve and blood vessel damage, as well as a greatly increased risk of heart disease.

More than 50 percent of insulin-dependent diabetics die of either heart or blood vessel disease. Part of the reason for this is that diabetes affects levels of cholesterol and triglycerides; another is that insulin-dependent diabetics have raised levels of a clotting agent in their blood. Until the 1980s, when it was shown that a high-fat diet is bad for the heart, diabetics were advised to follow a high-fat, low-carbohydrate diet. Diabetics are now urged to eat a diet that is high in fiber and low in fat and sugar.

Diabetes and ethnicity

In Western countries people of Indian, Sri Lankan, Pakistani, and Bangladeshi descent have an average of 40 percent higher mortality from coronary heart disease than those of European or other stock. One of the reasons may be that the incidence of diabetes is five times higher among south Asians than in Europeans. With a low-fat diet, this risk factor can be reduced.

PERSONALITY

In the 1950s two San Francisco doctors, Meyer Friedman and Ray Rosenman, developed a theory that a certain personality type was more susceptible to heart disease than others. They claimed that Type A individuals, who tend to be aggressive, competitive, and impatient, are more likely to develop heart problems than Type B individuals, who are more patient and easygoing.

Although the Type A and B classifications are no longer used because they were based on men with white-collar jobs and did not represent the general population, certain psychological characteristics, such as coping badly with stress, are associated with heart disease and considered to be important.

AGE

In both men and women, deaths from coronary heart disease increase with age. About three out of five people who die of a heart attack are aged 65 and older. However, aging alone has little effect on the risk of coronary heart disease. The age factor is primarily due to the cumulative effects of lifestyle risk factors. Over a lifetime the effects of smoking and raised blood pressure and cholesterol levels take their toll. Modifying these conditions in the earlier years may protect against developing heart disease later on in life.

IS YOUR HEART AT RISK?

This quiz is designed to tell you if you are at risk for coronary heart disease. Read each question carefully and be sure to answer honestly. Place a check in all the boxes that apply to you, add them up, and then see below for what your score means.

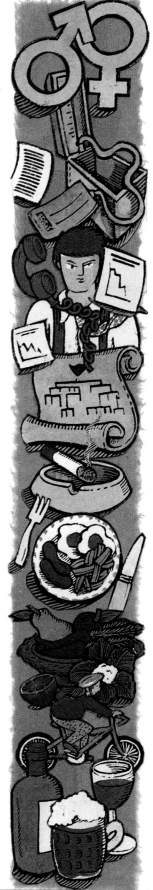

ARE YOU MALE AND UNDER 65?

If you are male, you are five to six times more likely to die in your forties from coronary heart disease than a woman of the same age. However, by the time women reach age 65, heart disease is the leading killer of women.

ARE YOU OVER 65?

Most heart disease occurs in people over 65, so the older you are, the more likely it is that you could be affected.

DO YOU HAVE A FAMILY HISTORY OF HEART DISEASE?

Doctors define a family history of heart disease as having a mother or sister who developed heart disease before age 65 and a father or brother who developed it before age 55. Such a family history is the single greatest risk factor for developing coronary heart disease.

DO YOU SMOKE?

Smoking cigarettes is the single greatest risk factor for coronary heart disease, after family history. Smokers at least double their risk of coronary problems.

DO YOU HAVE HIGH BLOOD PRESSURE?

High blood pressure, or hypertension, puts extra strain on the walls of your arteries, which can damage them, eventually causing a heart attack or stroke (see page 41). Blood pressure over 140/90 is too high.

ARE YOU OVERWEIGHT?

If you are more than 30 percent over the ideal weight for your height (see page 97), you are more likely to have raised cholesterol and blood pressure levels and to develop diabetes; you are at greater risk for heart disease.

DO YOU DRINK HEAVILY?

Heavy drinkers run a far greater risk of developing heart disease. Moderate drinking (up to two glasses of wine a day for a man or one for a woman) seems to lower the risk of heart attack compared to abstaining.

IS YOUR DIET HIGH IN SATURATED FATS?

Saturated fats are turned into cholesterol by the liver. Too much cholesterol can clog your arteries (see page 38).

DO YOU HAVE A RAISED CHOLESTEROL LEVEL?

A total cholesterol level of over 200 mg/dl greatly increases your chances of developing coronary disease. Doctors recommend that you keep your LDL level below 130 mg/dl and your HDL above 35 mg/dl. Very high levels of HDL actually protect against heart disease (see page 38).

IS YOUR DIET LOW IN FRUITS AND VEGETABLES?

You should be eating at least five servings of fruits and vegetables every day. They help your heart by providing antioxidant vitamins (A, C, and E), which help prevent LDL cholesterol from oxidizing and clogging arteries, and they are also a good source of water-soluble fiber, which can help to remove cholesterol from your body.

DO YOU HAVE A STRESSFUL JOB?

If your job is making you tense and irritable, it could raise your blood pressure. People who have little control over their working conditions are sometimes more stressed than high-powered executives.

DO YOU EXERCISE LITTLE OR NOT AT ALL?

People who are active have a 45 percent lower risk of developing heart disease. To strengthen your heart, you need to do at least 20 minutes of aerobic exercise three times a week (see page 71).

HOW DID YOU SCORE?
If you answered "yes" to fewer than six of these questions, you run a relatively low risk of coronary heart disease, but it is worth examining those questions to which you had a yes answer to see if you can lower your risk level further. If you answered "yes" to six or more questions, you should consult your doctor for advice on decreasing your risk.

AVOIDING HEART DISEASE

Heart disease can often be avoided by decreasing its risk factors. Quitting smoking, lowering blood pressure, and reducing cholesterol levels are three important measures.

The primary avoidable risk factors in coronary heart disease are smoking, high blood pressure, and high blood cholesterol. Having a combination of any two or all three is serious cause for concern. The more risk factors that individuals have, the more likely they will develop heart problems. A person who smokes and has high cholesterol levels and elevated blood pressure is eight times more likely to experience a heart attack than someone without any of these risk factors. Obesity, physical inactivity, and constant stress also contribute to a person's increased risk. They, too, should be dealt with.

THE EFFECTS OF SMOKING

Smoking is responsible for 3 million deaths a year worldwide. If the current smoking patterns continue, the toll will rise to about 10 million deaths by the year 2025. This gloomy forecast refers to deaths not only from lung cancer but from all tobacco-related diseases, including heart disease.

Major investigations have shown that smokers are at two to three times higher risk for developing heart disease than nonsmokers. The more cigarettes that people smoke and the more years they smoke, the greater the risk of having a heart attack.

Much of the evidence concerning the health risks posed by cigarette smoking was gathered in a landmark study from 1951 to 1971 by Dr. Richard Doll and Dr. Richard Peto of Oxford University. This study of the hazards of tobacco use in 34,000 British male doctors showed that about half of all people who smoke cigarettes regularly will eventually die as a direct result of their habit. It also showed that half of these will die prematurely in middle age, thus losing 20 to 25 years of life expectancy.

Many studies that have looked at the effects of giving up smoking have shown that the risk of developing heart disease falls quite rapidly as soon as a person stops the habit. But some studies have shown that it takes between 5 and 10 years after quitting for an ex-smoker to reduce his or her risk of

In the brain constriction of blood vessels can cause a stroke.

Nicotine from lungs passes to the brain and stimulates the sympathetic nervous system.

In the lungs carbon monoxide is taken up by red blood cells and reduces oxygen uptake.

Adrenal glands produce more adrenaline in response to nicotine.

Arm arteries become constricted by carbon monoxide and nicotine.

Sympathetic nervous system stimulates adrenaline production.

Heart rate increases because of adrenaline. Blood pressure also rises.

Leg arteries become constricted by carbon monoxide and nicotine. This may lead to muscle death and possibly require amputation.

SMOKING AND YOUR HEART
Smokers have a greater risk of heart disease and stroke than nonsmokers. The nicotine from smoking increases adrenaline production, causes constriction of artery walls, and increases the chance of blood clots. It also increases cholesterol buildup in coronary arteries, leading to atherosclerosis and high blood pressure.

coronary disease to the level of someone who has never smoked. All the studies agree that there is every good reason to stop smoking because it will undoubtedly decrease the risk of a heart attack, as well as improve general cardiovascular health.

Cigarette smoking and heart disease

Carbon monoxide and nicotine are the major substances in tobacco smoke that affect the heart. Nicotine, a highly addictive drug, stimulates the sympathetic nervous system (see page 21) and adrenal glands. This increases adrenaline production, makes the heart beat faster, and raises blood pressure. The rise in blood pressure, although temporary, may damage the arteries; there is evidence that smoking increases the buildup of fatty deposits in the arteries, or atherosclerosis. Nicotine also increases the risk of cardiac arrhythmias and spasm of the coronary arteries. Carbon monoxide bonds with the blood's red pigment, which is called hemoglobin. Once bonded, the capacity of the blood to carry oxygen to the heart is reduced. Both carbon monoxide and nicotine also encourage blood clotting, which can increase the risk of heart attack.

Passive smoking

Nonsmokers who live or work with smokers are at risk for lung cancer, but there is still some debate over whether passive smoking can cause heart disease too. A Chinese study of 200 people, published in the *British Medical Journal* in 1994, claimed to show for the first time that passive smoking is linked to heart disease. Researchers from Xi'an University found that nonsmoking women whose husbands smoked were more than twice as likely to develop heart disease than those with nonsmoking husbands.

How to quit

Because smoking is so habit forming, giving it up can be difficult. The most common reason smokers give for not quitting is that they are afraid they will get fat. Putting on weight, however, is not an inevitable consequence of stopping smoking. Your appetite may increase once you quit, but it is still possible to avoid weight gain by exercising more. Those who put on weight usually lose it within six months to a year of quitting.

There is no easy way to quit. The simplest method is just to stop; millions of people have done so without any special help. But some people find that going "cold turkey" is too difficult. They cannot cope with the withdrawal symptoms, which include inability to concentrate and nicotine cravings. The physical craving for nicotine can last from a week to several months.

To guard against starting to smoke again, it is important to recognize and consider how to deal with the times when the craving for a cigarette is likely to be greatest, such as when drinking alcohol or at times of stress (see page 36 for help on quitting).

Other quitting methods include joining a stop-smoking group. These groups can provide support and advice for people who find it difficult to quit on their own. Also available are nicotine chewing gums and nicotine patches. These can help, but the addiction to nicotine will still need to be confronted if you use these. Acupuncture and hypnotherapy can also be valuable aids in giving up cigarettes (see box, left).

Reduce or quit?

To avoid quitting, some people change their smoking habits instead, hoping to reduce their risk of heart disease. Cutting down does not reduce your risk significantly, nor does switching to cigars or pipes or to filter or low-tar cigarettes. Switching products will not lower the risk because cigarette smokers tend to inhale deeply and will do the same with other tobacco products.

The simple fact is that only giving up smoking completely can dramatically reduce an individual's chances of developing heart disease. It is the biggest single improvement to health a person can make.

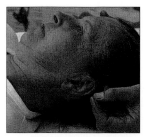

EAR ACUPUNCTURE FOR SMOKING
Needles are inserted into, or tiny metal balls are taped onto, pressure points in the ear for combating addiction.

Pathway to health

Some natural therapies can help you to quit smoking and also to cope with the psychological and physical effects of withdrawal.

Hypnotherapy is recommended for giving up the habit. While you are in a relaxed state of consciousness, the therapist plants suggestions in your mind about quitting smoking. It may take more than one session to be successful.

Another way to halt the addiction is with acupuncture. An acupuncturist applies standard needles to pressure points in your ear during a session or tapes tiny needles or metal balls over the pressure points and leaves them for a while.

Once you have stopped smoking, you can ease a cough and calm your nerves with an herbal infusion of red clover and valerian. Place 1 teaspoon each of the dried herbs in a cup of boiling water and steep for 10 minutes. Drink the tea several times a day. See an herbalist for other ways to reduce symptoms.

Quit Smoking

Smoking is an addiction in which there is a psychological as well as a physical dependency. It requires great determination and perseverence to break the addiction. Several techniques that can help you eliminate the habit are discussed below.

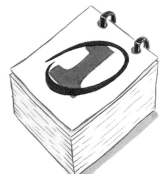

SET THE DATE
To help yourself prepare for quitting, decide on a day some weeks or months ahead of time and then stop on that day.

HUMMING MEDITATION

For some people, getting in the right frame of mind is simply a matter of spending time thinking about the benefits of stopping. To reinforce this process, consider using one or more forms of relaxation exercises, especially those that involve deep concentration on the result you desire. For instance, try meditating daily on your desire for a clean, healthy, smoke-free body. You can use self-hypnosis to the same end, or you can try deep breathing exercises, which will enable you to feel calm.

Letting go of any addiction or bad habit has to involve an emotional commitment. Sometimes it can take a long while to get in the right frame of mind, but for most quitting methods to work effectively, getting the mental attitude right is essential.

Increasing your ability to relax will help you prepare for quitting by reducing the levels of stress that compel you to reach for a cigarette.

An especially effective form of relaxation is humming meditation. For maximum benefit, practice it at the same time every day as part of your routine. Pick a place that is quiet and where you will not be overheard or disturbed. Wear loose clothing and sit in a comfortable position, either cross-legged on the floor or in a supportive chair.

Meditation can aid you in making your mental commitment to the process, after which you can use one or more other approaches to help maintain your quitting drive and prevent you from slipping back into the habit once you have stopped.

Before you begin the meditation, formulate an affirmation that you feel is appropriate for you: for instance, "I am no longer going to pollute my body with nicotine" or "I want my body to be clean, healthy and vital." Repeat this meditation once or twice a day or whenever you feel the need to have a cigarette.

Humming meditation yields positive results because the different tones and rhythms of humming induce a hypnotic state and are very soothing to the mind.

1 *Close your eyes and observe your breath going down, down into your abdomen and then up and back out again. Concentrate on the breath itself and gently push aside any intrusive or unwanted thoughts.*

2 *After six deep, slow breaths, allow yourself to hum on each exhalation. Choose any pitch you like for your humming and try to make the tone as long and drawn out as possible.*

3 *After a few minutes of humming, you should be feeling relaxed and calm. On each inhalation you can now repeat your affirmation in your mind. Continue meditating for 10 to 15 minutes.*

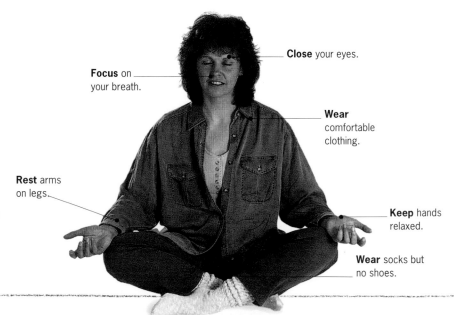

Focus on your breath.

Close your eyes.

Wear comfortable clothing.

Rest arms on legs.

Keep hands relaxed.

Wear socks but no shoes.

THE QUITTING PLAN

Pick a day a few weeks from now—Q-Day, when you will smoke no more cigarettes—and begin to prepare for this day. On Q-Day the break from cigarettes must be complete. Trying "just one" will take you straight back to smoking.

PREPARE YOURSELF

In preparation for Q-Day, try the methods below for making it easier to follow through with your plan.

Make a list of all the situations in which you usually smoke, including daily occasions and less common ones. Write down what you will do in each situation to avoid that particular cigarette. For example, instead of having a cigarette after a meal, leave the table and do the dishes.

Tell your friends, family, and work colleagues that you are quitting and ask for their support and patience.

Cut out the best cigarette of the day—such as the one on rising in the morning or with after-dinner coffee.

Make yourself conscious of every cigarette you smoke. Try putting a rubber band around the pack.

Smoke your first cigarette one hour later each day. Make a day-by-day graph of cigarette consumption to see the numbers falling.

Avoid very smoky places if at all possible. Try not to socialize with smokers during the first few weeks after you quit and ask your friends and family not to smoke around you. Go to places where smoking is not allowed, such as the movies.

Cut down on your intake of alcohol and caffeine. These substances are often mentally associated with smoking. Also, some research has suggested that they increase the craving for nicotine.

Read everything you can about the effects of smoking on your health.

THE DAY ITSELF

On the day you have assigned as your Q-Day, here are some things you can do to make it easier.

Get your teeth cleaned at the dentist. Wash all your clothes and bed linens; clean the carpets and your car; spray your house with air freshener; open all the windows and wash the curtains; throw away all ashtrays, matches, and cigarettes.

Remind yourself of all the reasons for giving up smoking, including that you will have a healthier heart and circulation, generally improved health, greater fitness, and better sexual performance. You will save money, enjoy the taste of food more, and have a better personal odor. Also, you will stop polluting the environment and affecting others with your smoke, especially children.

TROUBLESHOOTING

You are bound to run into a few problems in the days and weeks after you quit. Here are some ways to overcome them.

▶ *Coughing: This is common after quitting. Keep cough drops handy and drink herbal teas.*

▶ *Dry mouth: Drink water all day.*

▶ *Irritability: Meditate every day. Avoid caffeine. Take a warm bath. Have a massage. Exercise more.*

▶ *Constipation: Eat more fruits and vegetables for soluble fiber.*

▶ *Hunger: Snack on low-fat, low-calorie foods.*

LASTING THE DISTANCE

So you've made it to Q-Day and you've taken the plunge. Now what? The weeks ahead will be difficult while you weather cravings and withdrawal symptoms. You must take further steps to avoid being enticed back to your habit. If you do slip, don't feel that you are a failure. Simply excuse it as a mistake and then continue with the quitting plan. Make sure you meditate or listen to relaxation tapes daily to relieve the stress of withdrawal. Do visualization exercises, like imagining the nicotine flowing out of your body; visualize your lungs filling with healthy air. Sit in non-smoking sections of restaurants and keep your home smoke-free.

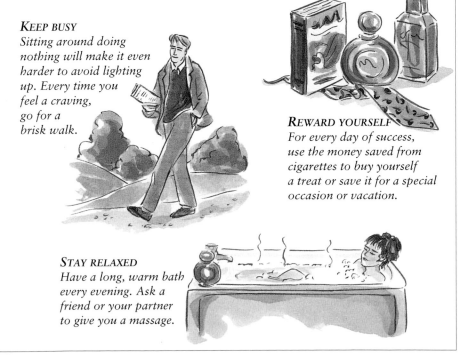

KEEP BUSY
Sitting around doing nothing will make it even harder to avoid lighting up. Every time you feel a craving, go for a brisk walk.

REWARD YOURSELF
For every day of success, use the money saved from cigarettes to buy yourself a treat or save it for a special occasion or vacation.

STAY RELAXED
Have a long, warm bath every evening. Ask a friend or your partner to give you a massage.

THE HEALTHY HEART DIET

Your daily diet should include at least five servings of fruits and vegetables and six servings of grain foods, such as rice, pasta, and bread. You should also

▶ *Choose cereal products that include bran, particularly oat or rice, for their fiber and cholesterol-lowering effects.*

▶ *Use nonfat or low-fat milk, yogurt, and other dairy foods instead of whole-milk products.*

▶ *Limit meat to a lean 3-ounce serving once a day or replace with a combination of legumes and cereals.*

▶ *Eat oily fish at least once or twice a week.*

▶ *Consume refined sugar and fat sparingly.*

DIET

The second important lifestyle risk factor after smoking is being greatly overweight. People who are obese, that is, have more than 30 percent body fat (see page 51), are more likely to develop heart disease than people of normal weight. Excess weight increases strain on the heart and influences blood pressure and cholesterol levels.

Growing evidence also suggests that the way fat is distributed over the body is important in predicting heart disease. "Apple-shaped" people, whose extra weight is mainly around their stomach, are at greater risk than "pear-shaped" individuals, whose fat is around the hips and thighs.

The fat factor

The recommendation for the general population is that total fat in the diet should be limited to 30 percent and saturated fat to 10 percent. People who have already suffered a heart attack or have other indications of heart disease, such as angina, should limit their fat intake even more. Many mainstream doctors, nutritionists, and alternative therapists now advocate a very low-fat, mostly vegetarian diet for heart patients.

Saturated fat is particularly bad for the heart because it increases not only total blood cholesterol levels but the "bad" LDL cholesterol that clogs arteries. This is the kind found in red meat, whole-milk dairy products, and other animal foods. Trans fatty acids, produced when vegetable oils are homogenized to make them solid at room temperature, are equally bad for the heart. These are found in stick margarines and baked goods made with hydrogenated fat.

Mono and polyunsaturated fats, the kind prevalent in most nuts, seeds, and certain vegetables, do not cause fatty buildup. In fact, monounsaturated fats, found in olive and canola oils, appear to reduce LDL cholesterol. (See pages 52–53 for more details on the different types of fat.)

CHOLESTEROL

Cholesterol is a fatlike substance made by the liver and carried in the bloodstream. Without it, the nervous system would not work properly. It is present in both blood and tissues and is an essential part of the cell walls, hormones, and bile salts of the body. In order to move around the body, cholesterol must be attached to lipoproteins (particles that are a combination of lipids, fat, and protein). There are two main types of lipoprotein: high-density (HDL) and low-density (LDL).

Good and bad cholesterol

HDL picks up cholesterol from the blood and takes it to the liver for processing or excretion. It actually removes the excess cholesterol from fat-saturated cells, including those of artery walls. HDL cholesterol is called the "good cholesterol" and actively protects you from atherosclerosis.

LDL, which carries 60 to 80 percent of the body's cholesterol, has a tendency to drop it in artery walls, causing plaques and atherosclerosis. It is important to know how much HDL cholesterol and LDL cholesterol you have, rather than just the total blood cholesterol, as this will indicate how healthy your heart and arteries are. (See page 52 for what different levels mean.)

Cholesterol levels

The level of cholesterol in the body is partly determined by genetic factors. Some people naturally have higher cholesterol levels. Anyone who suffers from familial hyper-

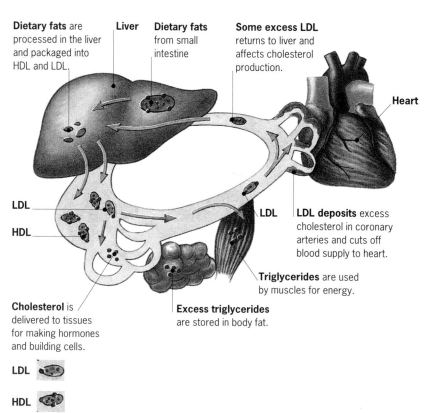

Dietary fats are processed in the liver and packaged into HDL and LDL.

Liver

Dietary fats from small intestine

Some excess LDL returns to liver and affects cholesterol production.

Heart

LDL

HDL

LDL

LDL deposits excess cholesterol in coronary arteries and cuts off blood supply to heart.

Triglycerides are used by muscles for energy.

Cholesterol is delivered to tissues for making hormones and building cells.

Excess triglycerides are stored in body fat.

LDL

HDL

lipoproteinemia (see page 32) have an abnormality in their genes that affects the way the liver handles cholesterol. As a result, their levels of blood cholesterol tend to be very high no matter what they eat.

Risks of high cholesterol levels

Elevated blood cholesterol is the most widely known risk factor for coronary heart disease. If the body has more cholesterol than it needs, this soft, waxy substance builds up in artery walls, making them narrower and thus slowing blood flow and eventually cutting off blood supply to the heart, the brain, or other vital organs. Virtually everyone, therefore, should try to maintain a diet that keeps their intake of cholesterol and saturated fat to a minimum.

Lowering cholesterol

To reduce cholesterol levels, you should substitute monounsaturated and polyunsaturated fats for saturated ones and reduce your fat intake overall.

Anyone who is overweight can lower blood cholesterol simply by dropping pounds. The only way to lose weight is to consume fewer calories than the body needs, so that fat stores are gradually used for energy. One way to cut down on calories is to eat fewer fatty foods and sugary foods like cakes and cookies.

ALCOHOL

Heavy drinking increases the risk of dying prematurely. Overindulgence in alcohol can lead to raised blood pressure, stroke, and cirrhosis of the liver. Moderate consumption, however, is not harmful. Indeed, there is evidence that it may have a protective effect on arteries (see page 64). It is thought that red wine in particular may protect against heart disease because it contains a substance that prevents LDL from being oxidized by free radicals (see page 58) and forming deposits in the arteries. Other types of alcohol are thought to be beneficial as well, because they interfere with the formation of blood clots that can block arteries.

It is recommended that men drink no more than the equivalent of two glasses of wine and women no more than one glass of wine per day. More than this moderate amount cancels the beneficial effects.

EXERCISE

Regular exercise is an important weapon in the fight against heart disease. More than 40 studies have confirmed the link between physical inactivity and a weakened heart. Overall, these show that inactive people have almost twice the risk of coronary heart disease as do active people.

How much exercise?

There is debate about exactly how vigorous and frequent exercise has to be before it starts to reduce the risk of heart disease, but it is widely accepted that to attain fitness, aerobic exercise (see page 71) should be done for a minimum of 20 minutes three times a week. In other words, it is better to do moderate exercise several times a week rather than strenuous exercise only once a week. This can range from brisk walking to intense aerobic dancing if you are fit.

Benefits

Exercise reduces blood cholesterol and high blood pressure and seems to help people relieve stress, all of which lower the risk of heart disease. It also encourages weight loss because the number of calories used by the body is increased during exercise, and regular exercise raises your metabolic rate, which continues at the elevated rate even when you are resting.

Types of exercise

Exercise can mean anything from sessions in the gym to square dancing to simply leading an active life. Vigorous housework or gardening, walking up stairs rather than using an elevator, and walking to the train station rather than driving can all contribute to reducing coronary risk. See chapter 4 for more details on exercising to strengthen the heart and improve circulation.

AEROBIC EXERCISE
An aerobics class is a convenient and enjoyable way to get some of your weekly exercise. It is important for your heart to be challenged for at least 20 minutes three times a week.

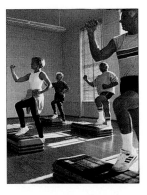

The stress tip-off

It is natural to feel stress as part of everyday life, but too much is bad for health. It is important to identify sources of stress and find ways to cope with them or lessen their impact. For instance, trying to see the positive side of a bad situation or laughing instead of giving in to anger can help relieve tension. Some psychologists recommend "acting as if you were happy," a practice that tends to dissipate negative feelings.

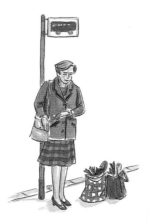

A SOURCE OF STRESS Waiting for a bus, in a bank line, or for the doctor can be stressful. But if you decide to view waiting as a pleasant opportunity to rest, to collect your thoughts, to read a book, or to perform a visualization exercise (see page 83), it will no longer be as stressful.

STRESS

All people experiences stress, although they may react to it in different ways. For example, a person who feels that life is one big struggle with no escape will have difficulty managing stress, as will someone who often feels angry and out of control. Such people may have health problems as a result. Individuals who approach life's ups and downs with a sense of challenge and purpose generally handle stress better.

Some scientists have noted a relationship between heart disease and the amount of stress in a person's life. For example, heart problems have been found to be higher among the recently bereaved and people in job sectors of high unemployment.

A theory developed in the 1950s by Meyer Friedman and Ray Rosenman (see page 32) pointed to the connection between personality and coronary heart disease, where the main component was an individual's susceptibility to stress. This has been modified and now centers around anger (see page 152). A 1994 study of 1,000 men who had had a coronary thrombosis found that they easily became annoyed and irritable.

Good and bad stress

Stress is natural and can often be useful, acting as a stimulant in challenging situations. "Good" stress, such as winning a contest, can be exhilarating. But stress becomes "bad" when you feel out of control, when everything is too much for you, when you believe life and people are against you, and when you are exhausted. This is the time to act (see page 146).

When you are feeling stressed, take into account that life circumstances may be contributing to it. Examples would be a change of house, job, or partner; the death of a loved one; financial problems; illness or injury. Write down exactly what is happening and how you can solve actual problems or improve your way of coping with them.

Reducing stress

It is important to deal with feelings of stress and anxiety as soon as possible. There are a number of methods that you can try.

Schedule your time reasonably. Write down a weekly timetable showing hours spent working, relaxing, exercising, and socializing. Try to develop interests outside of work. All work and no play is a bad idea.

It will be easier to exercise regularly if you schedule yourself an exercise routine that is varied in approach (see page 74). Try not to get too serious and competitive about it, though, especially if you include a team sport. Exercise should be fun and enjoyable, not an additional source of stress.

Practice relaxation techniques. Join a meditation class or buy some tapes. Try some visualization methods (see page 83) or simply listen to relaxing music in a peaceful environment. Consider treating yourself to a flotation tank (see page 83) or a massage.

For problems you cannot deal with yourself, seek assistance from a person who can, such as an accountant or a doctor. Or talk to a friend about your worries.

BLOOD PRESSURE

In order for blood to reach every part of the body, it must be propelled under pressure. The pressure caused by the heartbeat is the systolic pressure, the diastolic pressure occurs when the heart relaxes (see page 23).

Blood pressure variations

The upper limit of normal blood pressure in an otherwise healthy person is 140 systolic and 90 diastolic. However, a person under 30 years old would be more likely to have a reading of 120/80. These values are

CHECK LIST

Check the symptoms you experience when you feel stressed.

- ✔ *Diarrhea or vomiting*
- ✔ *Head, stomach, and/or back pain*
- ✔ *Dizziness, fainting, palpitations*
- ✔ *Loss of appetite and libido*
- ✔ *Overeating*
- ✔ *Depression, low self-esteem*
- ✔ *Worry and anxiety*
- ✔ *Anger, hostility, arguing a lot*
- ✔ *Trouble sleeping*
- ✔ *Fatigue*
- ✔ *Forgetfulness*
- ✔ *Skin rashes*

When you next have any of these symptoms, use relaxation methods to relieve them.

expressed in millimeters of mercury (see page 23). Blood pressure readings vary at different times of the day and during different activities. Blood pressure falls to lower levels when a person is sleeping and is elevated during times of stress. It also tends to rise overall with advancing age.

Blood pressure and pregnancy

Pregnancy can cause an increase in blood pressure. Normally, blood pressure falls during the first few months of pregnancy, then rises again in the later stages. High blood pressure, however, may also develop for the first time during pregnancy, a condition known as pre-eclampsia, which can develop into eclampsia, or toxemia of pregnancy. It occurs in about 15 percent of pregnant women but is most common in women over 35 and those who are having their first baby or are carrying more than one fetus.

Pre-eclampsia rarely causes complications if it is treated as soon as possible. One of the first signs of the condition is swelling of the face, feet, and hands, and there may be protein in the urine. Headaches, dizziness, and nausea may also be experienced if the condition remains untreated. The next stage is true eclampsia, in which uncontrollable seizures and coma occur.

Pre-eclampsia does not start usually until after the 20th week of pregnancy, but blood pressure may rise progressively before this time. It is vital, for a pregnant woman's pressure to be checked regularly. The condition is controlled with rest and sometimes blood pressure–lowering drugs. A patient may be admitted to a hospital for observation. In severe cases birth may be induced or a caesarean section performed.

Blood pressure and cardiovascular disease

People with untreated high blood pressure have a greater than normal risk of developing strokes and heart and kidney disease. If the blood pressure remains high over a long period, then the constant force of the blood through the arteries means they are more likely to be damaged.

Controlling blood pressure

Several factors play an important role in controlling blood pressure. If yours is high, you need to do everything possible to reduce it as soon as possible. If you are overweight,

EFFECTS OF HYPERTENSION

Hypertension, or high blood pressure, can cause damage to arteries in different areas of the body, including the brain, eyes, heart, and kidneys. High blood pressure also increases the risk of atherosclerosis, coronary heart disease, and stroke.

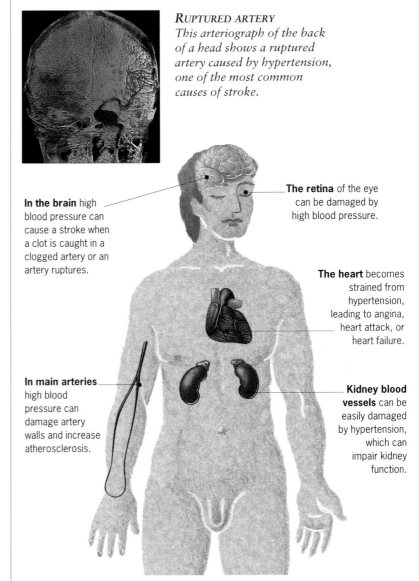

RUPTURED ARTERY
This arteriograph of the back of a head shows a ruptured artery caused by hypertension, one of the most common causes of stroke.

In the brain high blood pressure can cause a stroke when a clot is caught in a clogged artery or an artery ruptures.

The retina of the eye can be damaged by high blood pressure.

The heart becomes strained from hypertension, leading to angina, heart attack, or heart failure.

In main arteries high blood pressure can damage artery walls and increase atherosclerosis.

Kidney blood vessels can be easily damaged by hypertension, which can impair kidney function.

you should go on a weight loss program. This is often the only measure needed to reduce blood pressure. If you drink, then limit your consumption to no more than two glasses of beer, wine, or spirits per day (one if you are a woman). Reduce fat, especially the saturated kind, and use salt sparingly if you are salt sensitive (see page 51). Stop smoking immediately (see page 36). Develop mechanisms that can help you to deal with stress, such as learning relaxation techniques (see page 82).

Autogenic Training

A form of self-hypnosis, autogenic training (AT) is an effective and simple way of reducing tension and stress by inducing deep mental and physical relaxation. People who use autogenics regularly have improved health and resistance to disease.

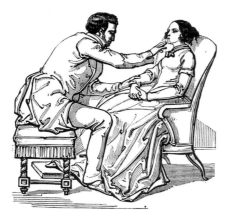

HYPNOSIS
Since the 1800s hypnosis has been used to treat various ailments. People often consult a hypnotist for help in quitting an addiction, learning to relax, or relieving pain. Those who respond well to being hypnotized will probably find autogenic training easy to learn and very beneficial.

Origins

Autogenic training as a system of self-hypnosis was developed by the German neuropsychiatrist Dr. Johannes Schultz in the 1930s. It was further developed and expanded by Dr. Wolfgang Luthe in Canada. The technique is widely employed today as an aid to relaxation and combatting stress. When practiced regularly, autogenics can be used to target the unpleasant effects of illnesses, as well as help people to get in touch with emotions. It can also help build creativity and enhance effectiveness in the workplace.

The principle behind autogenics training (AT) is "passive concentration," which fosters deep relaxation. Positive suggestions can then be introduced to reduce stress, change bad habits, or encourage creativity.

How do you learn autogenics?
The method is usually taught in a group of 6 to 10 students, and the sessions are normally given weekly for a period of 8 to 10 weeks. During this period students learn the basic relaxation techniques and how to apply them.

More advanced training includes the use of specific positive affirmations, or autosuggestions, and meditations to increase health, well-being, and energy levels. Although it is recommended that you attend classes to

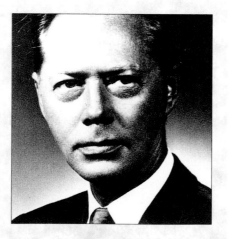

DR. WOLFGANG LUTHE
Luthe helped to develop the practice of autogenic training and introduced it to a large number of people.

obtain the best results, it is possible to teach yourself autogenics by following a carefully laid-out course of home study. In this case it is important to be disciplined, follow the instructions exactly, and not be tempted to accelerate the course or change the affirmations.

Where can I find a trainer?
There are private clinics that specialize in autogenics. The trainers are usually doctors, psychologists, nurses, naturopaths, or other qualified health care practitioners who have trained and received a certificate in the method.

What happens in the first session?
An autogenic trainer will give you a general checkup to make sure you can do the training safely. You will be asked questions about your medical history and personality. Anyone who has heart disease will be trained only under medical supervision.

A trainer will teach you the basics of autogenics in one or two sessions. You will choose a relaxing posture, and the trainer will talk you through the six basic exercises, or verbal formulas, asking you to visualize feelings of heaviness, such as "my left leg is heavy," feelings of warmth, for instance, "my right arm is warm." You will also focus on the heartbeat, warmth in the stomach, calming the breath, and coolness on the forehead.

You will be asked to visualize each of these conditions until every part of your body is relaxed. The trainer may then introduce some positive suggestions and affirmations that are tailored to your specific needs and problems.

How often should you practice autogenics?

Regular practice is essential; your trainer will probably recommend practicing three times a day initially; doing it morning, noon, and night is the ideal. The advantage of autogenics is that it can be done in any quiet location, as long as you remain uninterrupted. Any comfortable place is suitable. It is important to practice between sessions so that your trainer can monitor your progress and effectiveness.

How does autogenic training relieve stress?

An autogenic trainer teaches you how to achieve a relaxed state at will and to move with ease and fluency from a state of excitement to a state of relaxation so that the pains and strains built up by chronic stress will be released as quickly as they form.

However, you choose the moments when you want to destress. For most people a reaction to stress is partly physical and partly emotional. Because the effects of stress also occur in pleasant situations—for example, meeting a loved one or anticipating an exciting event— clearly the stress reaction is not always undesirable, and indeed many people find a certain amount of stress stimulating because it allows them to be more focused.

What problems respond well to autogenic training?

With practice you can learn how to formulate affirmations that are tailor-made to suit your needs. Autogenics is not a cure for physical problems, but attitude and emotions have been shown to be important in fighting disease. In this respect, autogenic training can enhance your immune system and help you tackle such problems as addictions, high blood pressure, palpitations, and persistent pain.

The method can be used in conjunction with other treatments as well. Consult your doctor or an autogenic trainer for further information on the compatibility of treatments.

How does autogenic training affect the emotions?

A release of stress will put you in touch with feelings that have been stored in the body, often as muscular tension. In autogenics, using a technique called offloading, accumulations of negative emotions can be released in a number of ways (see page 155). The trainer will teach you various vocal techniques—such as singing, screaming, moaning, or making baby noises—and physical techniques to release frustration, anger, and tension. Even sadness and anxiety may be offloaded this way.

Autogenics does not in any way deal with the analysis of emotion, and if negative feelings cannot be simply released using offloading, you are advised to seek counseling or psychotherapy.

WHAT YOU CAN DO AT HOME

Do this exercise as many times as possible during the day: the more, the better. Sit in a comfortable chair, hands palm down beside you or resting on your thighs, eyes closed.

Step 1: Slowly scan your body in your mind; start with the toes and move up the front, then the back.

Step 2: Concentrate on your dominant arm (right if you are right-handed, left if you are left-handed). Say, "My right (left) arm is heavy" and let your mind travel down its length. Your arm may become heavy, light, warm, or tingly or do nothing at all. Just be aware of it. Repeat the phrase three times. Do the same routine with your other arm.

Step 3: Clench both fists tightly and bend your elbows, then stretch your arms straight out in front of you. Inhale a deep breath, open your eyes, and breathe out. Repeat the second two steps three times.

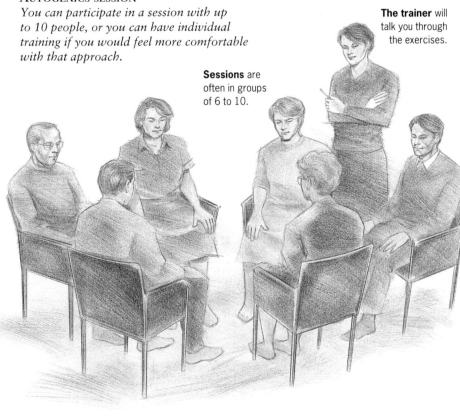

AUTOGENICS SESSION
You can participate in a session with up to 10 people, or you can have individual training if you would feel more comfortable with that approach.

The trainer will talk you through the exercises.

Sessions are often in groups of 6 to 10.

THE IMPORTANCE OF CHECKUPS

It is vital for individuals with a known high risk of heart disease to have regular checkups. This applies particularly to middle-aged and older people because the risk increases with age.

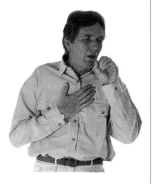

COUGHING
A bad cough can sometimes cause chest pain similar to angina.

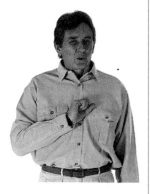

HEARTBURN
Pain in the chest from indigestion may be confused with heart-related chest pain.

People are often worried unnecessarily about various symptoms that they confuse with heart-related problems. One of the most common of these is "heartburn"—a feeling of burning in the middle of the chest—which is usually caused by indigestion and is treated with antacid tablets. Heartburn often occurs after eating and is made worse by spicy or fried foods.

Chest pain is also a cause for concern, but it can be the result of muscle strain or injury to the rib cage. Have you been in an accident, suffered a sports injury, or had a severe cough? Any of these could be causing chest discomfort. Heart palpitations (a rapidly beating heart) can occur when you are under extreme stress, feel fear or excitement, or drink a lot of coffee. Also, some common over-the-counter drugs, such as sinus tablets, contain a lot of caffeine, which can make your heart feel fluttery.

If you are in any doubt at all, you should seek medical attention (see page 86 for symptoms related to heart disease).

HAVING A CHECKUP

If heart disease is suspected, your doctor will do an extensive checkup. He or she will take a family history, look at your personal medical history, and do a complete physical examination. This usually includes measuring blood pressure, heart rate, and various pulses; checking veins for any swelling; listening to breathing and heart sounds (see page 20); taking a chest X-ray; and doing an electrocardiogram (ECG). Routine blood tests, for cholesterol and other lipid levels, blood cell counts, oxygen levels, and cardiac enzyme levels, may also be done (see page 90).

Depending on the results of this initial examination, the doctor may decide to send you for further tests in order to make a more definite diagnosis. These may be non-invasive ones, such as an exercise stress test, echocardiography, rapid computed tomography (CT) scanning, or magnetic resonance imaging (MRI), or more invasive tests, like cardiac catheterization. These and other tests are explained on pages 90–95.

Tell your doctor

For a checkup to be most effective, it is important that you give your doctor as much information as possible. Before you go for your appointment, think about the following and write down anything that you might forget when you arrive: all prior illnesses, accidents, and hospitalizations; any allergies (to medications, foods, and so on); any chronic illnesses, such as asthma; any medication you are taking (including the contraceptive pill); any unhealthy lifestyle habits, such as smoking or drinking heavily; any medical problems that run in the family, such as high blood pressure, high cholesterol, and heart disease; and any other relevant details. It is also vital that you discuss all symptoms that are bothering you and ask any questions you have.

You may decide after having a medical checkup that you would also like the opinion of a natural therapist (see page 99), such as a naturopath, homeopath, or traditional practitioner of Chinese medicine (who uses herbs and acupuncture). The above information is just as relevant to such therapists because they need to obtain a complete picture of you, your lifestyle, and your habits. They may also ask additional questions concerning your moods, emotions, relationships, sources of stress, and your reactions to different situations and circumstances.

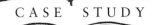

A Middle-aged Woman at Risk

As people approach middle age, they tend to put on weight because their metabolism slows down and they become less active. Being overweight and not getting enough exercise increases the risk of coronary heart disease, diabetes, and hypertension. Regular checkups are important to ensure that optimum health is maintained.

Alison, a 44-year-old accountant, is married to Jonathan, a lawyer. They have two teenage children, Tom and Sarah. Alison has just moved to a highly demanding job in a new partnership. When she is sent for a routine medical checkup, the company doctor tells her she is 10 kg (22 lb) above her ideal weight and her blood pressure is too high—150/95. The doctor suggests that she try to lose weight by adopting a healthier diet and getting more exercise on a regular basis.

Alison is worried about changing her lifestyle; she has always been too busy with work to exercise and take much notice of what she eats. Her husband and children similarly lead busy lives and, unfortunately, also have unhealthy eating habits.

WHAT SHOULD ALISON DO?

Alison's busy life leaves little time for shopping or cooking, let alone exercise. Alison needs to manage her time more effectively so that she can fit healthful eating and a regular exercise routine into her schedule. This will help her to lose weight, as well as to reduce her blood pressure and better control her stress levels.

Alison must learn about healthier foods and make an eating plan that is realistic for her lifestyle and that of her family. She needs to make changes in her diet, incorporating healthier snacks and well-balanced meals. She can get information about nutrition and exercise from her doctor or a dietitian. Bookstores and magazine stands also offer myriad publications on these subjects.

Action Plan

WORK
Organize work schedule more efficiently. Have a nutritionally balanced lunch every day and snack on fresh fruit. Park farther from work and walk.

FAMILY
Plan the family menu in advance and enlist family's cooperation in shopping and cooking to meet everybody's needs and desires. Include more fruits and vegetables.

LIFESTYLE
Cut down on own portion sizes. Buy an exercise bike and ride every evening for half an hour.

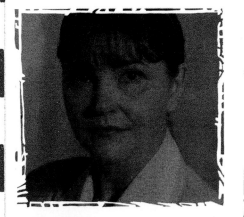

WORK
A high-pressure job and long working hours can leave you tired and stressed and result in poor lifestyle habits, such as eating on the run.

FAMILY
When the whole family is on the go constantly, poor eating habits may develop that can be difficult to change.

LIFESTYLE
Little exercise and a high-fat, high-sugar diet result in overweight and a higher risk for heart disease.

HOW THINGS TURNED OUT FOR ALISON

Alison and her family have established a shared shopping and cooking routine and now enjoy healthier eating. In three months Alison has lost 5 kg (11 lb) and feels more energetic. Her doctor says her blood pressure is normal. She is enjoying her job more because she does not feel so stressed and tired, and she is pleased to see her family becoming more health conscious. If she breaks her eating plan occasionally, she does additional exercise.

RULE OF THUMB FOR CHECKUPS

Until you reach 40 years of age you should have a physical checkup every three to five years, then four times during your forties and five times during your fifties. Annual examinations are advised for people over 60. It is important to go for additional checkups if

▶ *You are feeling unwell.*

▶ *You experience unusual symptoms.*

▶ *You drink heavily or smoke.*

▶ *You have a family history of heart disease, high cholesterol, or hypertension.*

▶ *You have diabetes.*

▶ *You are overweight.*

▶ *You are constantly under great stress.*

▶ *You are pregnant.*

STANDARD ECG
This test will be carried out on anyone who is suspected of having heart disease. It may be followed by an exercise ECG (see page 91).

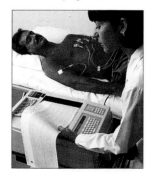

SCREENING POPULATIONS: REDUCING THE RISK

In the United States heart disease kills as many people as all other diseases put together. Cardiovascular disease is also the leading cause of death in Canada, but deaths account for 37 percent of the total. Health strategies to reduce the number of deaths aim to tackle the three major risk factors: smoking, high blood pressure, and high blood cholesterol.

Campaigns against smoking have reduced the number of deaths from heart disease in recent years, as people have become more aware of the effects of smoking. More public education about reducing cholesterol levels with a diet lower in fat, especially saturated fat, could lower the numbers further. Education in schools and the workplace is focusing on the importance of regular exercise, healthy eating, and avoiding smoking and heavy drinking.

Government health departments in the United States and Canada recommend that people know their cholesterol level by having regular checkups and then act on it, if necessary, by changing their diet. This is particularly advised for anyone with a family history of heart disease or who has diabetes or at least two of the following risk factors—obesity, high blood pressure, inadequate physical activity, and smoking.

CHOLESTEROL TESTING

Your doctor may decide to test your blood cholesterol levels when you go for a checkup, particularly if there is a family history of high cholesterol. Cholesterol tests may also be done during other screening checks, such as for breast cancer.

It is possible to buy home-testing cholesterol kits if you are interested in monitoring your own level (see page 96).

A high reading does not necessarily mean that a heart attack is just around the corner. Your doctor will be able to balance the cholesterol measurement against other factors to properly assess your personal risk level. He or she will be able to advise you on changes you should make to your lifestyle and diet to minimize the chances of heart problems in the future.

BLOOD PRESSURE TESTING

Family doctors should routinely check blood pressure, especially if other risk factors for coronary heart disease are present. Adults should have their blood pressure checked at least once every three years. Women who are on the contraceptive pill should also have their blood pressure measured whenever they receive a new supply.

One high reading does not mean that you have high blood pressure; levels fluctuate at different times of the day and under varying circumstances. Therefore, to get a true picture of blood pressure levels, it is important to take a measurement after sitting quietly for a few minutes. If the level is high, your doctor may take your blood pressure again at the end of your appointment. If it is still high you will be advised about further action. Home blood pressure measuring kits are available (see page 96), although these are not quite as accurate as the ones used in a doctor's office.

ELECTROCARDIOGRAPHY

Electrocardiography is the most commonly used test to diagnose heart disease. A machine records the electrical activity of the heart when electrodes (gel pads) are attached to each arm and leg and to six places on the front and left side of the chest. The test is painless and harmless.

The trace produced is called an electrocardiogram (ECG). It shows if there are any abnormalities, but sometimes it may suggest there are problems even when the heart is perfectly healthy (see page 91). Further tests can be done to confirm or rule out a particular diagnosis (see pages 93–95).

Stress test

In many patients with heart disease there are no symptoms at rest, and an ordinary ECG is normal. But exercise may bring on changes in an ECG, so an exercise ECG, or stress test, is sometimes used to diagnose heart problems, especially angina.

The patient exercises either on a treadmill or a stationary bicycle. The test usually takes about 15 minutes and ECG readings are taken both during and after the exercise routine (see page 93).

CHAPTER 3

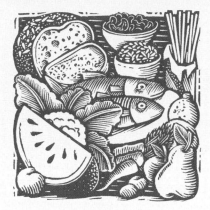

EATING TO PROTECT YOUR HEART

"You are what you eat" is a phrase with particular relevance to heart disease. About 30 percent of people who die from this condition do so because of their diets. Since heart disease develops gradually over many years, it is best to establish good eating habits at an early age and follow them throughout life. But even changes made later in life can have a beneficial effect on the heart. Diet is one of the major "natural" weapons in the fight against heart disease.

DIET AND HEART DISEASE

The commonsense, well-balanced diet that protects against cancer and obesity is equally effective at lowering the risk for heart and other cardiovascular diseases.

Medical researchers have looked at the eating habits of people in different countries to try to establish a connection between food and heart disease. The results are now well documented.

THE DIET CONNECTION

Many earlier links between diet and heart disease were based on The Lipid Hypothesis, first proposed by an American professor, Ancel Keys, in the 1950s. (Lipids are fatty compounds, which include fats, fatty acids, carotenoid pigments, cholesterol, and oils.) Professor Keys found that many populations whose diets were high in fat had a higher incidence of heart disease than those with a lower fat intake. A high fat intake, especially of the saturated kind found in meat and dairy products, was linked to elevated blood cholesterol levels. Further studies during the 1970s and 80s showed that a high blood-cholesterol level was one of the most important risk factors for heart disease.

As a result, there is now an increased focus on healthier cooking methods and greater intake of foods that seem to offer some protection against heart disease. There is evidence, for example, that it is not just a lower fat intake in Japan, China, or the Mediterranean countries that results in a lower rate of heart disease, but it's also the amounts and types of other foods that these people eat. Based on such findings, many experts have put forward recommendations to help reduce the rate of diet-related diseases, particularly heart disease.

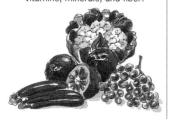

Fresh produce provides plenty of heart-protecting vitamins, minerals, and fiber.

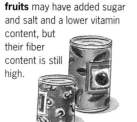

Frozen foods usually retain most of their nutrients if they are frozen correctly.

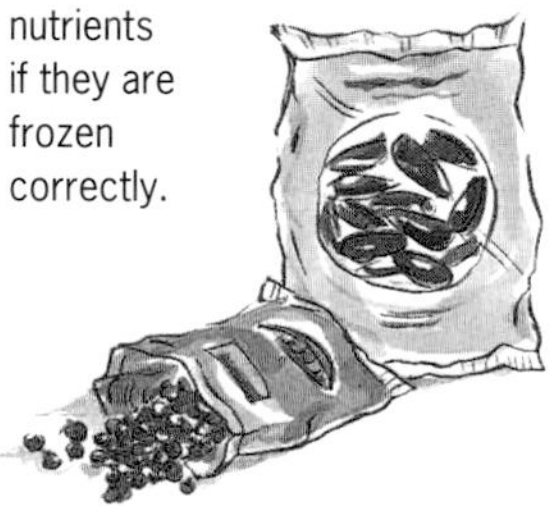

Canned vegetables and fruits may have added sugar and salt and a lower vitamin content, but their fiber content is still high.

FOCUS ON FOOD
Eating at least five servings of vegetables and fruits every day—fresh, frozen, or canned—helps protect the heart.

HEART DISEASE AND THE MEDITERRANEAN DIET

The rates of death from heart disease (per 100,000 people) and fat intake (as a percentage of total calorie intake) for different countries around the world are given in the chart to the right. The most striking fact revealed by this chart is the relationship between the low-fat, high-fish, and high-vegetable diet of the Japanese and their low rate of heart disease compared to that of Western countries. However, the highest fat intake is for Greece (48 percent of total calories), yet the rate of heart disease in that country is well below the rate in Finland (with only 37 percent). This and a similar result for France and Italy has been attributed to the special effects of the "Mediterranean diet" (see page 56).

COUNTRY	CORONARY HEART DISEASE *	FAT INTAKE **
Scotland	779	40
Finland	629	37
England & Wales	595	40
United States	454	45
Germany	381	47
Greece	287	48
Canada	272	38
Italy	252	41
France	133	46
Japan	77	31

* Death rate per 100,000 population
** Percentage of total calorie intake

Eating for a healthy heart

Most people in the Western world eat too much fat; it constitutes about 40 percent or more of their total calorie intake. Since fat plays a key role in the development of heart disease, experts now recommend reducing overall fat intake to 30 percent or less of total calories (see page 53 for how to calculate your fat target). Recommendations also include eating less saturated fat, prevalent in animal foods like meat and whole-milk dairy products, and trans fatty acids, created by hydrogenation of vegetable oils.

The backbone of any diet should be complex carbohydrates, such as bread, potatoes, rice, pasta, and low-fat, low-sugar breakfast cereals. These foods should make up about half of your daily calorie intake and form the main part of all your meals and snacks. To obtain the fullest benefit from the vitamins and minerals found in these foods, choose the varieties that are highest in fiber, such as brown rice and whole-grain breads and cereals. The dietary fiber in these foods is also important because it helps lower elevated blood cholesterol levels.

Fruits and vegetables also play a key role in the prevention of heart disease. Current guidelines call for at least five servings of fruits and vegetables every day. Fresh or frozen ones are best; the canned varieties can be high in sugar and salt (check the labels) and rarely have the same level of vitamins and minerals because of the processing necessary to preserve them. Also, include the skins of apples, potatoes, and other fruits and vegetables as often as possible for their fiber content.

Other suggestions for a healthy-heart diet include eating oily fish one to three times a week, regularly including nuts and seeds in the diet, reducing salt intake, and drinking only moderate amounts of alcohol.

Developing good eating habits

Putting the advice of the experts into practice can be difficult when it comes to food. Most people eat for a number of reasons other than being hungry or trying to stay healthy. Food provides pleasure and helps to ward off boredom and depression.

Changing to a healthy eating pattern may take some time and organization, so it's best to make changes gradually rather than all at once. Start by eating at least three regular meals a day, including breakfast. If possible,

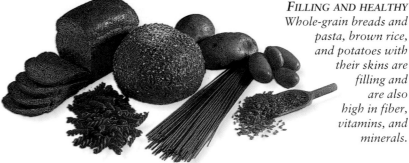

FILLING AND HEALTHY Whole-grain breads and pasta, brown rice, and potatoes with their skins are filling and are also high in fiber, vitamins, and minerals.

have your main meal in the middle of the day, when you need energy, and only a light meal in the evening. Eat as wide a variety of food as possible and in moderate portions, following the dietary guidelines recommended on page 62.

Avoid skipping any meals; you may become so hungry later that you can't resist unhealthy snacks. It is all too easy to reach for foods like potato chips, cookies, and candy, which are high in fat, salt, and/or sugar. Such foods can be eaten occasionally as a treat, but should not make up a major portion of anyone's diet because they provide so little nutritional value. Eating regularly also helps control body weight. Studies show that many overweight people tend to skip meals, often compensating with high-calorie snack foods.

Some people prefer to "graze," eating smaller meals at more frequent intervals. As long as the foods chosen are healthy ones, this pattern of eating is fine. Eating more frequently can also help prevent overeating as a result of being too hungry.

HEALTHY CHOICES

Light meals and between-meal snacks should be low in fat and sugar. Always choose low-fat or nonfat dairy products and mayonnaise; also use fresh produce whenever possible. Eat margarine and butter sparingly or not at all.

Fresh fruit mixture with low-fat yogurt

Baked potato with low-fat cottage cheese and vegetables

Walnuts, hazelnuts, and pecans

Chicken breast sandwich

Crackers with low-fat cheese, tomato, and cucumber

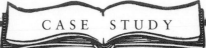

A Gourmet Traveler

Adopting a healthier eating pattern is challenging enough when you are at home. But people whose work requires extensive travel and dining with clients and business colleagues in restaurants may find the prospect even more daunting, especially when health concerns indicate that a radical change in diet is necessary.

Chris is a 48-year-old civil engineer who works for a large construction company that carries out projects all over the world. He spends approximately 70 percent of his time overseas, which suits him because he has always loved good food and wine and he enjoys the opportunity to try out the cuisines of many different countries.

At his last annual company checkup he learned that he had a high cholesterol count, which alarmed him because he has a family history of heart problems. The doctor advised him to cut down on fatty foods. Chris does not have a sweet tooth and is only a moderate drinker. He works out at least three times a week at hotel health clubs and he swims regularly.

WHAT CHRIS SHOULD DO

Chris must cut down significantly on his fat intake. He should eat less French food because it is often rich in cream, butter, and eggs, and more Italian food, selecting low-fat pasta dishes and excluding the creamy sauces, of course. Middle Eastern cuisine offers healthy meals based on grains and vegetables. Japanese food is another good choice, with its emphasis on rice and lightly-cooked and raw vegetables, fresh fish, and few dairy products. He should also eat less meat and avoid using fatty spreads, like butter or margarine.

Because he doesn't like sweets, Chris usually ends his meal with cheese. He should cut back on this practice. Better still, he should eat some fruit instead.

Action Plan

EATING PATTERNS
Do not skip breakfast. Eat fresh fruit or juice, whole-grain cereal or bread, and low-fat yogurt. Choose oatmeal for a hot breakfast. Limit eggs to four a week.

WORK
Try to choose restaurants where there are some low-fat dishes on the menu. If there is no choice, be extra careful the next day.

DIET
Cut down on meat. Eat more poultry, fish, and vegetables. Choose low-fat or nonfat dairy products. Avoid fried foods and creamy sauces and dressings.

EATING
Starting the day with a healthy and satisfying meal reduces the temptation to snack later on.

DIET
A diet that is rich in meat and dairy products and low in fruits and vegetables can cause a high cholesterol level.

HOW THINGS TURNED OUT FOR CHRIS

Chris kept a diary to monitor his consumption of saturated fats and to list restaurants that offered foods more suitable to his new diet. After trial and error with ways to cut fat and still enjoy food, he successfully reduced his saturated fat consumption. By his next medical checkup Chris had lost 3 kg (6½ lb) and his cholesterol was at a healthier level, but he realized that he would have to remain vigilant to ensure that it did not climb back up again.

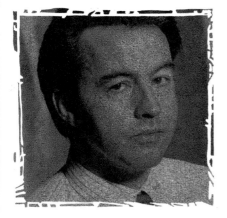

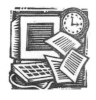

WORK
Business dinners in a foreign country can make it difficult to stick to a healthful diet.

ARE YOU OVERWEIGHT?

One way to calculate if you are overweight is to use the Body Mass Index (BMI): your weight in kilograms (kg) divided by height in meters (m) squared. (To convert pounds to kilograms, divide by 2.2; to convert inches to meters, divide by 39.37.)

For example, for a woman whose height is 1.6 m (63 in) and weight is 62 kg (136 lb), the computation is: 62 divided by (1.6 x 1.6) = 24.2

A BMI of 20 to 24 indicates a healthy weight; between 25 and 30 is considered overweight; and over 30 is obese. A BMI below 20 indicates underweight and this too can cause some health problems. Though it is a helpful indicator, the BMI should be used as a guideline only because build and age must be taken into account. Consult your doctor.

Obesity

Maintaining a healthy weight is important because being overweight doubles the risk of developing heart disease. With more than half the adults in North America (more than 100 million people) now classified as overweight and 23 percent as obese (30 percent over their ideal body weight), it has become increasingly vital for people to reduce their weight to more healthful levels.

Obesity increases the risk of heart disease because it is linked with raised blood pressure and blood cholesterol levels. Also, too much body weight overworks the heart. And if you are carrying a lot of extra weight, you will be less likely and probably less able to exercise. Many overweight and obese people develop diabetes, which also has been linked to an increase in the risk of early heart disease (see page 32).

Beware of diets

Although weighing a healthy amount is desirable, it is important not to become obsessive about what you eat. Any positive dietary changes need to be followed long-term. Going overboard on any diet usually causes failure because the diet places too many restrictions and makes it impossible to lead a normal life. A new diet should be practical and fit in with the way you live. Also, sudden dietary changes can cause fluctuations in magnesium and potassium levels that may affect your heart's normal rhythm.

AVOIDING HIGH BLOOD PRESSURE

Raised blood pressure is a well-known risk factor for heart disease because it can cause damage to arteries that supply the heart muscle. It usually does not have a single cause—several factors, including diet, play important roles—but in people who have moderately high blood pressure, dietary changes are often enough to keep the condition under control.

High blood pressure is particularly common in overweight people. Losing excess pounds and maintaining a normal weight usually helps reduce blood pressure.

Heavy drinking also raises blood pressure. A modest intake of alcohol may do no harm and may actually be beneficial, but too much can be dangerous (see page 119).

People with high blood pressure who are sensitive to sodium must greatly limit their salt intake. For most patients, however, doctors advise a moderate reduction, which can be achieved by not adding salt when cooking; tasting food before adding salt; using herbs and spices for flavor instead; and cutting down on processed foods. Over time, taste buds gradually adjust to a low-salt diet and people find they do not miss it.

Potassium, an electrolyte that helps maintain the body's normal balance of salt and fluids, helps keep blood pressure normal. Most fruits and vegetables contain some amount of this mineral, but bananas, citrus fruits, avocados, dried apricots, legumes, whole grains, tomatoes, and potatoes are particularly rich sources.

Many experts also recommend that people who have high blood pressure reduce their intake of fatty foods, both to help lower blood pressure and to reduce the overall risk of heart disease.

CAUTION
Too much potassium can be harmful for people who have kidney problems or are on certain kinds of medication. A potassium salt substitute should be used sparingly and with a doctor's approval.

PROCESSED FOODS

Many ready-cooked or packaged foods are high in salt (sodium chloride) and should be avoided or used sparingly by people with high blood pressure who are sodium sensitive. They include:

▶ *Processed meat, such as bologna, ham, bacon, salami, and sausage.*

▶ *Smoked meat and fish and meat and fish pastes.*

▶ *Canned foods, unless the label specifies "No added salt."*

▶ *Salted chips, pretzels, popcorn, and nuts.*

▶ *Most cheeses.*

▶ *Condiments, like olives and pickles, and bottled sauces, like ketchup.*

▶ *Soup stocks, bouillon cubes, and gravies.*

▶ *Packaged meals.*

THE PINCH TEST
If you can "pinch an inch" of fat on your waist, you probably need to lose some weight. Check the weight chart on page 97. Consult your doctor before embarking on a weight-loss program.

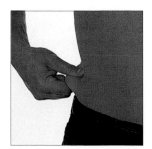

FATS AND HEART DISEASE

A heart-healthy diet is limited both in total fat and saturated fat, to keep blood cholesterol levels down and decrease the possibility of building up dangerous fatty deposits in arteries.

Different fats

The saturation of a fat is determined by the amount of hydrogen bonded to its carbon atoms. When a pair of carbon atoms is free, that is, not bonded to hydrogen atoms, a double bond forms between them.

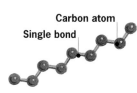

Carbon atom
Single bond

SATURATED
The carbon atoms are all bonded to as many hydrogen atoms as possible.

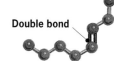

Double bond

MONOUNSATURATED
All carbon atoms are bonded with hydrogen except one pair, which forms a double bond.

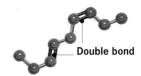

Double bond

POLYUNSATURATED
Several pairs of carbon atoms are free and joined by double bonds.

Atherosclerosis, or hardening of the arteries, occurs when plaque made up of fatty material is deposited on the inside of arterial walls. This condition is caused, in part, by excess fat in the diet.

DEVELOPMENT OF HEART DISEASE

There is plenty of evidence that clogging of arteries with fatty deposits begins during childhood. Once plaques have formed, they continue to grow, making the inner layer of the artery wall thicker and less elastic. The buildup of plaque causes the channel of the artery to narrow and restrict blood flow; this in turn raises blood pressure and puts a strain on the heart as it tries to force blood through the narrowed arteries. Plaque can also cause inflammation in blood vessels, which increases the risk of heart attack and stroke by promoting thrombosis, or clot formation (see page 125). Atherosclerosis may take 20 to 30 years to develop to the point where it produces symptoms. Unfortunately, the first sign of the condition is often a fatal heart attack.

The role of cholesterol

Early research into links between dietary fat and blood cholesterol levels looked at the incidence of heart disease in different countries and considered the effect of the local diet. Raised blood cholesterol levels were implicated in an increased risk for atherosclerosis and thrombosis.

Cholesterol is carried in the blood mainly by two types of proteins, called lipoproteins; these are high-density lipoproteins (HDLs) and low-density lipoproteins (LDLs). Yet a third type, very-low-density lipoproteins (VLDLs), carry a small amount of cholesterol, as well as triglycerides, another lipid.

Less efficient at carrying cholesterol, VLDLs and LDLs tend to drop some of it in the arteries, where it builds up as plaque. HDLs, on the other hand, collect cholesterol from arteries and other tissues and transport it to the liver, where it is metabolized and eliminated from the body. People with high levels of LDL and low levels of HDL are usually at high risk for heart disease.

In a typical cholesterol screening, the total amount is measured. A reading of 200 milligrams per deciliter (mg/dl) or lower is desirable. When the total is higher than 200 mg, levels of LDL and HDL are then measured separately. LDL levels should be below 130mg/dl; 130 to 159 is borderline high; and above 160 is classified as high. HDL levels should be at least 45 mg/dl, and higher is considered better.

In assessing caradiovascular risk, doctors also calculate the ratio of total to HDL cholesterol by dividing total cholesterol by the HDL figure. For example, if your total cholesterol is 220 and your HDL is 50, your ratio is 4.4. A desirable ratio is less than 4.5, so you would be in a lower-risk category. The best ratio is below 3.5.

TYPES OF DIETARY FAT

Fluctuations in blood cholesterol level are due mainly to the amounts and types of fat in your diet. There are three types of fat in food: saturated, monounsaturated, and polyunsaturated. The differences lie in their chemical bonding. The carbon atoms in saturated fats are linked by single bonds because the other bonding sites contain hydrogen; those in monounsaturated fats have one double bond; those in polyunsaturated fats have more than one double bond. The last two contain fewer hydrogen atoms and are liquid at room temperature, but they can be made solid by adding hydrogen atoms, a process known as hydrogenation.

Fatty foods contain different combinations of all three fats, with one fat predominating. Most animal foods are high in saturated fat; the fat in plant foods, except coconut, palm, and palm kernel oils, is largely unsaturated.

A high intake of saturated fat tends to raise LDL cholesterol levels because saturated fat is turned into cholesterol by the liver. The general recommendation is to limit saturated fats to 10 percent of total calorie intake. But many experts say that the ideal percentage is actually lower.

Monounsaturated fats
These fats are liquid at room temperature and solid when refrigerated. When they constitute the majority of fat in the diet, the level of HDL is increased and the level of LDL reduced. To protect your heart, monounsaturated fats should be the main fat in your diet. The best sources of monounsaturated fats are olive oil, canola oil, avocados, and most nuts.

Polyunsaturated fats
These are also liquid at room temperature and remain liquid when refrigerated. They tend to reduce total cholesterol levels but do not increase the "good" HDL levels. Many vegetable oils, including sunflower, corn, safflower, soybean, and cottonseed oils, are high in polyunsaturated fats.

Two polyunsaturated fats, linoleic and linolenic acid, are deemed "essential" fatty acids. They are not only necessary for growth, regeneration of tissues, and normal metabolic processes, but they also appear to protect against autoimmune diseases, cancer, and heart disease. Neither of these fatty acids can be made in the body so it is important to obtain them in your diet.

Omega-3 fatty acids
Fish, especially oily fish like mackerel, tuna, herring, and sardines, are excellent sources of omega-3 fatty acid, derived from the essential linolenic fatty acid. Nuts and seeds, especially walnuts and flaxseeds, are good plant sources. A high intake of omega-3 fats promotes a reduction in the stickiness of blood platelets and the tendency of blood to clot, as well as lowering triglyceride levels, all of which can reduce the risk of a heart

YOUR DAILY FAT TARGET
To maintain a healthy heart, you should limit total and saturated fat intake each day to the amounts indicated in the table below, or even less. (To determine your calorie limit, see page 142).

CALORIE LIMIT	TOTAL FAT INTAKE (grams)	SATURATED FAT INTAKE (grams)
1,000	30	10
1,200	40	12
1,500	45	15
1,800	55	18
2,000	60	20
2,500	75	25
3,000	90	30

All figures are rounded off.

attack. Studies show that people who have had one heart attack and subsequently increased their intake of omega-3 oils have reduced the likelihood of having another one. Experts recommend eating fish at least once and preferably two or three times a week and/or a tablespoon of flaxseed oil daily.

Although omega-3 oil is available in capsules as a supplement, it should never be taken without the advice of a doctor. It can be dangerous when used by heart patients who are on a regimen of aspirin or another blood-thinning agent.

Trans fatty acids
Trans fatty acids occur when mono or polyunsaturated fats are hydrogenated to make them solid at room temperature. They are found in stick margarines, shortening, and many processed foods, such as cookies, cakes, and fried foods, prepared with hydrogenated fat. It appears that trans fatty acids are even worse than saturated fats in terms of raising LDL and lowering HDL levels and thus increasing the risk of heart disease.

Since it became known that trans fatty acids can be harmful, some manufacturers of margarine have developed products that contain few or no trans fats. These are available as soft, or tub, style margarines; their labels usually state that they are low in trans fats.

Triglycerides
Three fatty acids and one glycerol (a type of alcohol) molecule make up the triglycerides, which transport the fat-soluble vitamins (A, D, E, and K) in the blood and help the body

IMPORTANT FAT
Oily fish is a good source of omega-3 fatty acids. These are believed to protect the heart by preventing clots.

If you do not eat fish, you can get omega-3 fats in rapeseed (canola) oil, flaxseeds and flaxseed oil, walnuts, and evening primrose oil; the last is available in capsules.

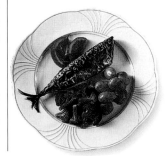

Measuring food energy

The energy value of food is measured in calories, but because one calorie is so small, figures are usually given in units of 1,000 calories, called a "kilocalorie" (kcal). This unit is also written as "Calorie," but "calorie," with a lower-case c, is now often used to mean kilocalorie, as it is in this book.

store energy. High levels of triglycerides are believed to increase the risk of heart disease because they play a role in blood clotting. Elevated levels are more common in overweight people, diabetics, alcoholics, and women taking oral contraceptives.

REDUCING FAT IN THE DIET

To determine if you are eating too much fat, you can calculate your daily fat target (see page 53) and then monitor how much fat you eat each day. You may have to reduce both total fat and saturated fat in your diet.

While some fats are visible, such as those in meat, cream, and butter, many are hidden in processed foods like cakes, cookies, potato chips, and chocolate. However, food products in the United States must state on the label the amount of total fat, saturated fat, and unsaturated fat in each serving, so it

is easy to check the fat content. In Canada, such information is sometimes available.

All salad and cooking oils contain about 14 grams of fat and 120 calories per tablespoon; butter, shortening, and stick margarines have 12 to 13 grams of fat and 100 calories per tablespoon; whipped butter and margarine contain 8 grams of fat and 65 to 70 calories per tablespoon.

By reducing the amount of fat you use in cooking it is possible to make a major impact on total fat intake. Healthy cooking practices (see Fat Savers, opposite), like straining fat off sauces and soups, trimming all visible fat from meat, and steaming or poaching food, help reduce fat in the diet. You can also use nonstick pans, which allow you to cook without any fat, or use nonstick cooking sprays, which enable you to cook with minimal oil.

FATS IN DAIRY FOODS

Some dairy products, like butter and heavy cream, are very high in saturated fat and should be used sparingly, if at all. However, dairy foods are an important source of calcium and high quality protein. To obtain these benefits you can choose from a variety of low-fat dairy products that give you the goodness without the fat.

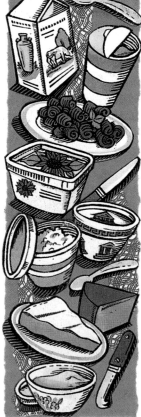

DAIRY PRODUCT 100 gram (3½ ounce) serving	SATURATED FAT in grams	MONO-UNSATURATED FAT in grams	POLY-UNSATURATED FAT in grams)	TOTAL FAT * in grams
Skim milk	0.06	Trace	Trace	0.1
Low-fat (1%) milk	1.0	0.5	Trace	1.6
Whole milk	2.4	1.1	0.1	3.9
Light cream	11.9	5.5	0.5	19.1
Heavy (whipping) cream	24.6	11.4	1.1	39.3
Light sour cream	6.6	1.0	0.1	8.25
Butter	54.0	19.8	2.6	81.7
Stick margarine	14.28	24.9	24.9	78.5
Soft (tub) margarine	10.7	10.7	21.4	49.9
Light spread (margarine)	0	12.5	18.7	37.2
Plain low-fat yogurt	1.0	0.4	0.2	1.7
Plain whole-milk yogurt	1.7	0.7	0.1	3.0
Large-curd cottage cheese	2.8	0.6	0.5	4.0
Low-fat cottage cheese	0.9	0.4	Trace	1.4
Cheddar cheese	21.7	9.4	1.4	34.4
Parmesan	18.9	7.7	0.4	31.5
Stilton	22.2	10.3	1.0	35.5
Cream cheese	19.4	9.0	0.9	31.0
Neufchâtel (cream) cheese	13.2	5.8	0.6	19.8

* Where the total fat quantity is more than the sum of the fats listed, the difference is trace quantities of other kinds of fat, including trans- fatty acids.

CHOOSING HEART-HEALTHY FOODS

Although it is generally easier to buy and eat processed or ready-made foods, they are often high in fat and salt and lower in nutrients. For a healthy heart, prepare as many meals as you can using fresh and natural foods and add little salt or sugar.

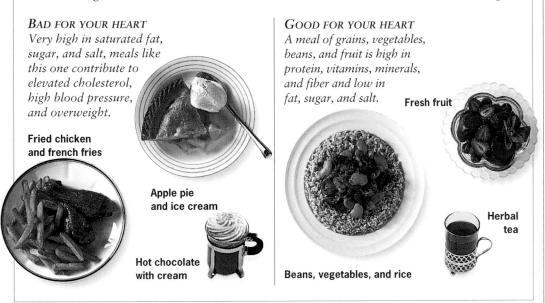

BAD FOR YOUR HEART
Very high in saturated fat, sugar, and salt, meals like this one contribute to elevated cholesterol, high blood pressure, and overweight.

Fried chicken and french fries

Apple pie and ice cream

Hot chocolate with cream

GOOD FOR YOUR HEART
A meal of grains, vegetables, beans, and fruit is high in protein, vitamins, minerals, and fiber and low in fat, sugar, and salt.

Fresh fruit

Herbal tea

Beans, vegetables, and rice

Low-fat dairy products

Whole-milk dairy products contain large amounts of both total and saturated fat. On average they contribute at least 20 percent of most people's total fat intake. However, dairy products are important because they are major sources of protein, iron, calcium, and other vitamins and minerals. Calcium is especially significant in controlling high blood pressure. You can still benefit from all these nutrients but avoid too much fat by choosing nonfat and low-fat versions. Select nonfat or 1-percent low-fat milk; the latter contains less than half the fat content of whole milk. Because young children need more fat than older youngsters and adults, they should be given only whole milk until they are at least five years old.

Choose low-fat rather than whole-milk yogurt, which is ideal to use in sauces, on baked potatoes, for extending mayonnaise and other salad dressings, and for topping fruit or a dessert. (Low-fat and nonfat sour creams are also available but do not contain calcium.) Avoid coffee creamers, which are often high in both total and saturated fat.

Whole-milk cheeses should not be eaten in large quantities, although, if you eat little meat, 60 grams (about 2 ounces) of whole-milk cheese three or four times a week will not push your saturated fat intake over the limit. Avoid cheese after a meal; you do not need the additional fat and calories if your menu has been balanced. Low-fat soft cheeses and cottage cheese can be substituted for the higher-fat variety the rest of the time, although cottage is low in calcium.

Low-fat high-protein foods

Meat and poultry are major sources of saturated fat. However, like dairy products, meat is also a valuable source of protein, vitamins, and minerals. To reap these benefits with less of the fat, you can choose lean cuts of beef, pork, and ham or eat chicken or turkey breast (the leaner part of the bird) without the skin. Eat sausage, bacon, salami, goose, duck, and heavily marbled steaks, which are very high in fat, infrequently. Always trim any visible fat from meat and add only minimal amounts of fat when cooking. When basting chicken, for example, use low-sodium stock instead of butter.

The best approach is to eat meat in smaller portions and less often. Many people have servings of 170 to 230 grams (6 to 8 ounces), whereas 85 to 115 grams (3 to 4 ounces) is sufficient. It is not necessary to eat meat every day, either. You can substitute poultry, fish, or a dish of grains and legumes for red meat at least four times a week. You will not miss large

LEAN MEATS
Except for an occasional special treat, choose lean cuts of meat and trim off any visible fat.

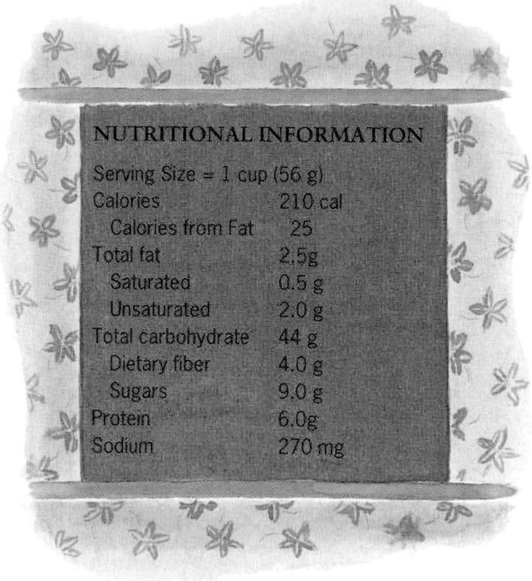

NUTRITIONAL INFORMATION

Serving Size = 1 cup (56 g)	
Calories	210 cal
Calories from Fat	25
Total fat	2.5g
Saturated	0.5 g
Unsaturated	2.0 g
Total carbohydrate	44 g
Dietary fiber	4.0 g
Sugars	9.0 g
Protein	6.0g
Sodium	270 mg

READING FOOD LABELS
Labels list nutritional information per serving, as well as the number of servings per package or container. Included also (though not shown here) are the vitamins, minerals, and cholesterol contained in a serving, plus the percentage of daily value (based on a 2,000 calorie diet) each number represents. You can compare the figures for different brands of a particular food to find the healthiest option.

helpings of meat as much if you fill out meals with more vegetables and such starchy foods as bread, potatoes, rice, and pasta. A little meat goes further than most people think because its complete protein enhances the incomplete protein in plant foods.

Reading food labels

There has been a massive increase in manufactured foods and ready-made meals over the last 25 years. Because such products are often high in fat, it is better not to eat them regularly. However, if you do use convenience foods, you can choose those that are more healthful by reading the labels.

In the United States food manufacturers are required by law to show a breakdown of nutritional contents, an example of which is shown above. Such nutritional labeling is voluntary in Canada, but when included, it must follow a standardized presentation similar to that used in the United States. (Books that list the nutritional contents of many common foods are also available.) Labels list not only the breakdown per serving but also the number of servings per container. You can decide how much of the food you will eat, then calculate how the food fits in with your daily fat targets (see page 53). The simple way to calculate the percentage of fat in a serving is to divide serving fat calories by serving calories. In the product, left, for example, the percentage of fat calories in a serving equals 12 (25 divided by 210). In a daily menu this food would balance another that is higher in fat.

Labels can help you select foods that have low total-fat and saturated-fat contents. They can also be helpful in finding low-fat alternatives to such products as breakfast cereals and salad dressings. But remember, the term "reduced fat" does not necessarily mean low fat. Reduced-fat potato chips, for instance, can still contain a great deal of fat, so you should eat small quantities only.

The Mediterranean diet

Many of the recommendations for eating for a healthy heart are already a natural habit in the southern European countries that border the Mediterranean, including Italy, Spain, and Greece. These countries share a common pattern of eating, which features large amounts of starch—bread, rice, and pasta—as a staple, plenty of fresh fruits and vegetables, and small quantities of meat, fish, and dairy products.

Most of the fat in the Mediterranean diet comes from olive oil, which is high in monounsaturated fat (the kind that raises levels of "good" HDL cholesterol). These Mediterranean countries all report a much lower incidence of heart disease than the countries of northern Europe and North America. Experts believe that many of the health differences are due to dietary factors and recommend that other countries adopt some of the positive aspects of the Mediterranean diet to reduce the incidence of heart disease.

MEDITERRANEAN-STYLE EATING
Adopting a Mediterranean diet means eating plenty of fresh fruits and vegetables, complex carbohydrates, and legumes, and the occasional glass of red wine.

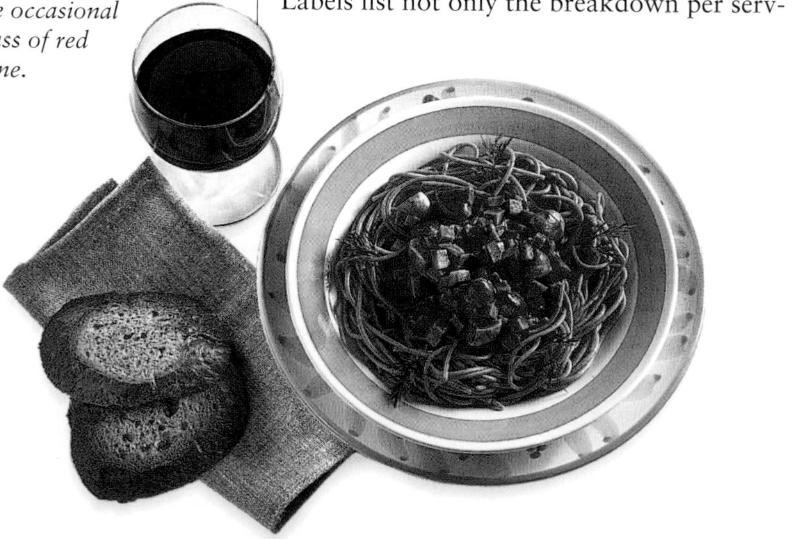

DID YOU KNOW?
Even if your diet includes no fat, your body will convert any excess calories from protein and/or carbohydrates into fat and store it as adipose tissue. Fat cells expand as additional fat accumulates. The fat cells of an obese person may be 50 to 100 times larger than those of a thin person.

CAUTION WITH FAT

You should not try to cut fat out of your diet completely because a small amount is needed for good health. However, it is important to use more unsaturated fats than saturated ones.

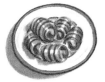

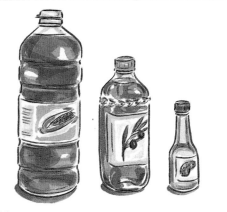

BUTTER
Butter contains largely saturated fat (54 percent), and should be used sparingly. Also limit red meat, cheese, palm and coconut oil, and cocoa butter (found in chocolate).

MARGARINE
Use margarine made from mono- and polyunsaturated fats and look for those that are low in trans fatty acids. Some newer tub margarines can even cut cholesterol levels.

OILS
Monounsaturated and polyunsaturated oils are recommended for salads and cooking. Monounsaturated oils include olive, peanut, sesame, and canola. These can actually lower LDL, or "bad" cholesterol levels and raise HDL levels. Polyunsaturated oils include corn, soybean, safflower, and sunflower. These will lower LDL cholesterol but not raise HDL levels, and they contain essential fatty acids.

Enjoy your food
No one should ban any food from his diet forever unless he is allergic to it. But for the sake of good health it doesn't hurt to eat some foods more often and others less often or sparingly. Every meal should include something that you really like, even if it's just a smidgen of butter on your toast or some toasted nuts atop your vegetables.

Also, make time in your daily schedule to sit down and relax while you are eating; you will digest your food better, be more aware of what you are eating, and enjoy it more.

Changing to a Mediterranean diet means eating more fruits, vegetables, grains, and legumes, moderate amounts of dairy products, fish, and poultry, and only small quantities of red meat. It also calls for using olive or canola oil as the main fat for cooking and salad dressings, and drinking the occasional glass of red wine with meals, unless your doctor advises otherwise. (People who do not drink at all are not advised to take up drinking. But benefits similar to those of wine can be obtained by eating grapes, especially red ones, and drinking red grape juice.)

Those who support the Mediterranean diet believe it can help protect against heart disease, as well as other diseases such as cancer, because of the particularly high quantity of protective antioxidant vitamins, A, C, and E, and of flavonoids and monounsaturated fat (see page 53). This concept is also used to explain the paradox of the French diet.

The French paradox

Like the southern Mediterranean countries, France has a lower reported incidence of heart disease than the rest of Europe. This has been puzzling to scientists because the French diet is actually high in saturated fats from butter, cheese, and cream.

This paradox of high total and saturated fat intake combined with a low heart disease rate is attributed by some experts to the presence of certain other foods in the diet. The French, like the southern Mediterraneans, eat a lot of the fruits and vegetables that are full of antioxidants. They also tend to drink red wine with meals, which has been shown to raise HDL cholesterol levels. (Red wine contains more antioxidant substances than white wine and may be more beneficial to the heart.)

The French paradox has made the discussion of diet and heart disease more complex as scientists realize that eating less fat or more unsaturated fat, although important, is not the whole answer. It appears that certain nutrients either promote heart disease or help protect against it. Therefore, numerous factors must be considered when suggesting a diet that is best for the heart. In addition to eating less of some foods, you need to eat more of others, particularly fruits and vegetables.

The way in which meals are eaten in France and the Mediterranean countries may also play a role. Good food is considered a deserved pleasure in these places, and eating with family and friends is an important part of life. Wolfing down a meal at an office desk, in a car at a drive-through restaurant, or in front of the television set may have effects beyond the actual nutritional value of the food. It might set the stage for heart trouble.

Saturated fat and cholesterol
Most cholesterol in your blood is actually made in the body from saturated fats you eat. The amount of dietary cholesterol has relatively little effect on the cholesterol level in healthy people. So when you buy a food product, check to see that it is low in saturated fat, not just low in cholesterol. And remember that only animal foods contain cholesterol, not plant foods..

FOODS FOR A HEALTHY HEART

Antioxidants and fiber are two key dietary elements that help keep the heart functioning at its best. Both of these are abundant in fruits and vegetables.

Better beta carotene
Beta carotene is the pigment in brightly colored fruits and vegetables that is converted to vitamin A in the body. Unlike other vitamins, beta-carotene is more available from cooked foods than raw ones. Cooking breaks down the chemical structure and releases the beta carotene. Shredding food does the same.

Important protectors against heart disease are the antioxidant vitamins and minerals, which help protect against the harmful effects of free radicals, oxygen molecules that damage body tissues.

FREE RADICALS
Every cell in your body needs a steady supply of oxygen to convert digested food into energy. But burning oxygen releases free radicals, unstable molecules that can damage healthy cells as they move through the body. Free radicals contain at least one unpaired, or negatively charged, electron, which makes them highly reactive. As soon as they are produced, free radicals start searching for positively charged molecules with which to react, or oxidize. An excess of free radicals can cause problems over time by setting up a chain reaction of destruction that damages cellular DNA and other genetic material. This destruction is believed to be a major factor in the aging process.

Metabolic processes are not the only sources of free radicals. They can come from elements in the environment, including industrial chemicals, air pollutants like auto exhaust, pesticides, the sun's ultraviolet rays, radon, and tobacco smoke.

Under normal circumstances the body has an elaborate defense mechanism, consisting of various enzymes, to control the buildup of free radicals and to prevent the tissue damage they cause. Antioxidants also play a major role in this defense.

ANTIOXIDANTS
Free radicals play an important part in the development of atherosclerosis by reacting with "bad" (LDL) cholesterol. In a 1992 study the U.S. National Institutes of Health and the Atherosclerosis Research Laboratory at the University of Mississippi found that giving people antioxidant vitamins raised "good" HDL cholesterol and reduced LDL cholesterol, thus lowering the incidence of atherosclerosis and heart disease.

The antioxidants are vitamins A (whose precursor is beta carotene), C, and E and the minerals selenium and zinc. There are many other plant chemicals, called phytochemicals, that may also help prevent cell damage and disease. These include bioflavonoids (the pigment in most fruits and vegetables) phenolic acid, isoflavones (found in legumes), tannins, and lignans (found in fatty fish, flaxseeds, and walnuts).

High-risk and low-risk diets
According to a 1994 study by the World Health Organization, both men and women in Glasgow are at a very high risk of heart disease compared to those in the rest of the world, with local women having a higher

FREE RADICALS

Free radicals damage tissue by adding oxygen to cells. The damaged cells then become free radicals. Free radicals may also act on cholesterol and cause atherosclerosis.

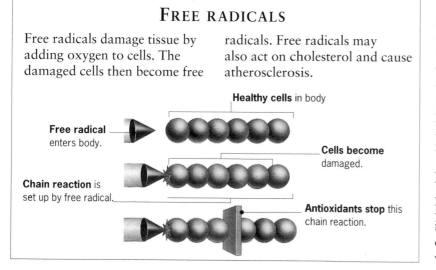

Free radical enters body.

Chain reaction is set up by free radical.

Healthy cells in body

Cells become damaged.

Antioxidants stop this chain reaction.

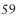

risk of dying from it than people in other regions. Factors such as smoking, obesity, lack of exercise, heavy alcohol intake, and high cholesterol are implicated, but residents also eat few fruits and vegetables, and high rates of heart disease are linked to a diet low in fruits and vegetables.

It is a long recognized fact that vegetarians suffer less often from heart disease than meat eaters do. This may be because they tend to have healthier lifestyles. But many researchers believe that their lower risk is probably due not only to avoiding meat but also to eating more foods that are high in antioxidants. Following this assumption, it may not be necessary to give up meat entirely but to eat less of it and substitute more of the foods that vegetarians eat.

Where are antioxidants found?

Except for vitamin A, which is found in fish, liver, egg yolks, and fortified milk products, the antioxidants are most abundant in fruits, vegetables, nuts, and seeds. (See box, below, for good sources of antioxidant vitamins.)

The World Health Organization recommends an intake of at least 420 grams (15 ounces) of plant foods every day, including 30 grams (1 ounce) of legumes, nuts, and seeds. Because it is difficult to translate this quantity into what goes on the plate, and it is impractical to weigh every morsel you eat, health experts recommend eating "five a day"—at least five servings of about 70 grams (2½ ounces) each of fruits and vegetables. To make sure you are getting these five helpings, you can include canned and dried fruit and fruit juices and frozen and canned varieties of vegetables, in addition to fresh ones. But keep in mind that many canned products have added salt and sugar, and they are often lower in nutrients. You should also include nuts and seeds, which are good sources of vitamin E.

MAGNESIUM AND POTASSIUM

Magnesium and potassium play significant roles in maintaining a healthy cardiovascular system; deficiencies are often associated with arrhythmias. The best sources of magnesium are leafy greens, whole-grain cereals, and legumes, so people who rely largely on processed foods may not be getting enough. Potassium is most abundant in bananas, avocados, citrus fruits, legumes, and whole-grain cereals (see also pages 51 and 141.)

BIOFLAVONOIDS
Although the role of bioflavonoids—the natural pigments of fruits and vegetables—in human nutrition is still being studied, some experts believe they are important for good health.

▶ *Many are thought to act as antioxidants and to enhance the antioxidant effects of vitamin C.*

▶ *Some are natural clot inhibitors.*

▶ *Many are believed to be involved in proper capillary functioning.*

▶ *A particular bioflavonoid in grape skins may be the ingredient in wine that reduces the risk of heart attacks among moderate wine drinkers.*

ACE FOODS

The antioxidant vitamins are A (whose precursor is beta carotene), C, and E. Foods containing them should be included abundantly in your daily diet. Doctors advise dietary intake rather than supplements because some antioxidants, taken in large amounts, may have the opposite effect and actually increase oxidation.

Beta carotene sources include carrots; dark green leafy vegetables, like spinach and broccoli; tomatoes; sweet potatoes; red, yellow, and orange peppers; mangoes; apricots; and cantaloupe.

Vitamin C sources include citrus fruits; strawberries; kiwi fruit; papaya; potatoes; green leafy vegetables; peppers; and broccoli.

Vitamin E sources include vegetable cooking oils, especially sunflower, soy, and corn oil; wheatgerm; whole-grain cereals; some green vegetables; almonds and other nuts; and most seeds.

EASY WAYS TO OBTAIN FIBER

If you follow the recommendation to eat at least five or six servings of whole-grain cereals and breads and five servings of fruits and vegetables each day, you will take in enough fiber. If you find this difficult, follow these suggestions.

▶ *Sprinkle oat or rice bran on breakfast cereal or yogurt.*

▶ *Each time you feel the urge to snack, eat a piece of fresh fruit, preferably with its skin.*

▶ *Eat the skin of potatoes, cucumbers, and other vegetables.*

FIBER AND HEART DISEASE

Fiber, or roughage, plays a part in protecting your heart. Fiber is the part of food that is not digested or absorbed by the body. There are two main types: soluble, which dissolves in water and becomes sticky, and insoluble. Both are found only in plant foods, and many plants contain both types.

Insoluble fiber—the two most common types are cellulose and lignin—is found in bran; whole-grain breakfast cereals and bread; nuts; asparagus, brocolli, and other vegetables; and the skins of fruits. This type of fiber is important in preventing constipation because it holds water in the bowels, making stools softer. It does not seem to have any effect on blood cholesterol levels or the prevention of heart disease.

Soluble fiber, found in many vegetables and fruits, rice and oat bran, and legumes, helps reduce total blood cholesterol and LDL cholesterol levels. Diets rich in soluble fiber are now often recommended as part of a cholesterol-lowering plan. However, eating lots of soluble fiber will not compensate for a high-fat diet. To reduce cholesterol levels effectively, total fat intake must be reduced and intake of fiber, especially the soluble type, must be increased.

If you are not used to eating fiber, you should introduce it into your diet gradually. Consuming too much too soon can cause abdominal discomfort, diarrhea, and flatulence because it ferments in the intestine. Increasing your fiber intake slowly gives your body a chance to get used to it and process it more efficiently.

How soluble fiber helps your heart

Soluble fiber is thought to help lower blood cholesterol levels by interfering with the absorption of fats and bile acids in the small intestine. Cholesterol binds to the fiber and is excreted with it. Fiber may also affect cholesterol metabolism in the liver.

Bile acids are made from cholesterol by the liver and released into the intestine to aid digestion of fats. Many of these cholesterol-heavy bile acids are reabsorbed into the blood and used again. The presence of soluble fiber breaks this recycling process and enables removal of cholesterol from the blood so it can be excreted. This process can lead to a reduction in total cholesterol and "bad" LDL cholesterol.

Fiber is also beneficial to diabetics because it slows down the absorption of nutrients in the blood, reducing blood sugar swings and

HOW FIBER WORKS

Soluble fiber helps reduce blood cholesterol levels by preventing the absorption back into the blood of some of the fats and bile acids in the small intestine. Instead, these fats are carried to the large intestine to be excreted.

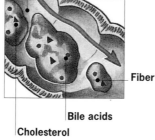

Large intestine

Fiber

Bile acids

Cholesterol

DIETARY FIBER
Although fiber is important for regulating the function of the intestines, the human digestive system does not possess the enzymes that are needed to break down fiber into an energy source. It therefore passes through the system virtually unchanged.

Cholesterol and bile acids are produced in the liver.

Fats and bile acids containing cholesterol are usually absorbed in the small intestine.

Fiber passes through the large intestine, taking cholesterol and bile acids with it to be excreted.

SOURCES OF FIBER

The two main types of fiber, soluble and insoluble, are found in different plant foods. Insoluble fiber is beneficial to your digestive system, while soluble fiber can help lower blood cholesterol levels, thus reducing the risk of heart disease.

INSOLUBLE FIBER
Excellent sources are whole-grain breakfast cereals and bread, brown rice, and whole-wheat pasta.

SOLUBLE FIBER
The best sources are fruits, vegetables, oatmeal, and dried legumes like lentils.

What about garlic?
Many studies have investigated the benefits of garlic. They show that fresh garlic and the extracts in enteric-coated garlic capsules and tablets help reduce total blood cholesterol, raise the level of "good" HDL cholesterol, and reduce the risk of blood clots, the usual cause of a heart attack. Garlic also lowers blood pressure in some people. A beneficial daily dose appears to be at least 10 milligrams of alliin, the active ingredient in garlic, or one to two raw cloves.

A note of caution: garlic pills should not be taken without first consulting a doctor because they may increase the effects of aspirin and other anti-clotting drugs, which can result in serious bleeding.

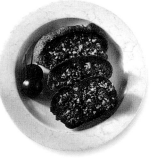

GARLIC TOAST
Try this Italian way of eating garlic . Toast some crusty bread, drizzle it with a little olive oil, and top with crushed garlic and minced fresh herbs.

the need for insulin. It is beneficial as well to people who are trying to lose weight because it is both filling and low in calories.

How much fiber do we need?

A healthy diet should include between 20 and 35 grams of fiber per day. You could obtain this from a daily intake of 3 tablespoons of oat or rice bran added to various foods, such as cereal or yogurt, rather than taken all at one time. However, a healthy diet should provide sufficient fiber. There is no need to count grams; simply eat lots of fruits, vegetables, legumes, and whole grains.

Drinking plenty of water—at least six to eight glasses a day—is important because fiber absorbs water and passes more easily through the digestive system. Consuming a great deal of fiber without sufficient water can cause bloating and gassiness. So, too, can increasing the amount of fiber in the diet too quickly. Eating too much bran and other foods containing insoluble fiber can also be a problem because certain substances in them bind with minerals like zinc, magnesium, iron, and calcium, decreasing their absorption by the body. Fiber supplements, which contain no other nutrients, are also likely to cause mineral deficiencies.

Is oat bran still a good bet?

For a study at the University of Kentucky in 1990 either oat bran or beans were added to the diets of people who had high blood cholesterol levels. Their total cholesterol was reduced by an average of 19 percent.

Two conclusions were drawn from this research. One was that such a massive reduction could be attributed in part to the large quantities of beans and oats eaten by the volunteers and the consequent reduction in other forms of food, as well as to the fact that the study involved people whose cholesterol levels were particulary high, making possible a greater drop. The second was that oats are a useful cholesterol-lowering food when part of a balanced low-fat diet. Further research has now confirmed a direct link between the amount of soluble fiber eaten and reduction in cholesterol.

Many people might not be able to eat enough oats to reduce their cholesterol levels drastically, but eating smaller quantities over a long period of time is beneficial. It is even better, however, to obtain soluble fiber from a variety of sources, including fruits and vegetables, to ensure that you get the benefit of other nutrients as well.

The Heart Diet

Some foods can help in the fight against heart disease, while others contribute to the problem. It pays to make a habit of eating more of the foods that protect your heart and fewer of those that may harm it.

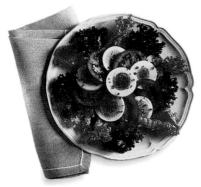

EGGS
Though four whole eggs a week is a recommended maximum, you can eat as many egg whites as you like; they are low in fat and cholesterol and high in protein.

No food is either good or bad, but the amount you eat of each one can make a difference. If your daily diet includes a variety of foods from the main groups shown in the pyramid below and in the amounts indicated, you will obtain all the nutrients you need to stay healthy. (For meal ideas, the sample weekly menu, opposite, offers a balanced and varied selection.) The keys to healthful eating are variety, moderation, and balance.

THE FOOD GUIDE PYRAMID

The pyramid here is an approximation of the one devised in 1992 by the U.S. Department of Agriculture (USDA) to help people remember the basics of healthful eating. Canada's Food Guide is similar but divides food into four basic groups with these daily recommendations—grain products, 5 to 12 servings; fruits and vegetables, 5 to 10 servings; milk products, 2 to 4 servings; and meat and alternatives, 2 to 3 servings.

Fatty and sugary foods
Eat oil, margarine, butter, chocolate, and pastries sparingly. Use mainly unsaturated fats.

Protein foods, including meat, fish, dried legumes, and nuts
Eat 2 to 3 servings totaling 170 g (6 oz) daily, but limit red meat and nuts. Poultry, beans, and oily fish are best.

Milk and dairy products
Eat 2 to 3 servings of low-fat dairy products (children under age 5 need whole milk). One serving equals 8 oz (1 cup) of milk or yogurt; 45 g (1½ oz) of cheese.

Fruits and vegetables
Eat 3 to 5 servings of vegetables and 2 to 4 servings of fruits. One serving equals 1 medium- size apple, ½ cup of diced fruit, ¾ cup of fruit juice,1 cup of leafy greens, ½ cup of cooked vegetables.

Starchy foods
Eat 6 to 11 servings of bread, cereals, pasta, and rice (in the UK potatoes are also included), preferably whole-grain varieties. One serving equals 1/2 cup of cooked pasta or rice, 1 slice of bread, 28 g (1 oz) of dry cereal.

A WEEKLY MENU

This menu has been created to give you an idea of what constitutes a wholesome and balanced eating plan. You can add low-fat snacks and additional beverages like herbal tea or coffee. Vegetarians can substitute legumes or tofu for fish or meat. As much as possible use low-fat dairy products and whole-grain varieties of bread, pasta, and rice. Choose breakfast cereals that are low in fat and sugar and canned fruit prepared in juice, not syrup.

	BREAKFAST	LUNCH	DINNER
MONDAY	Whole-grain cereal with sliced banana and skim milk; one slice whole-grain toast with low-sugar jam or jelly	Sandwich of grilled vegetables and feta cheese on cracked-grain sourdough bread; grape juice	Stir-fried chicken with broccoli, onions, and mushrooms; steamed brown rice; sliced strawberries topped with low-fat plain yogurt
TUESDAY	Half a cantaloupe; oatmeal with raisins or dried cranberries and skim milk; one slice whole-grain toast with soft margarine	Salad of lettuce, hard cooked egg, tomatoes, cucumbers, peppers, and olives; two slices whole-grain bread; bunch of grapes	Lentil soup with whole-grain roll; grilled vegetable kebabs; couscous; stewed fruit topped with low-fat custard
WEDNESDAY	Cranberry juice; one poached egg; two slices whole-grain toast with soft margarine; glass of skim milk	Corkscrew pasta salad with sliced chicken breast, tomatoes, olives, and sesame seeds; apple	Beef chili or beef stew; corn bread; salad of watercress, green onions, and cucumber; low-fat fruit yogurt
THURSDAY	Half a grapefruit; bran cereal with raisins and skim milk; two slices whole-grain toast with low-fat cream cheese	Two small baked potatoes filled with tuna salad, chili, or shredded low-fat cheese; orange juice	Pasta with artichoke hearts, tomatoes, onions, and garlic; baked apple
FRIDAY	Orange juice; 2 whole-grain toaster waffles topped with warm stewed apples or all-fruit jam; glass of skim milk	Salad of chickpeas, avocado, onion, and tomatoes on two whole-wheat pita breads; dried apricots or figs	Poached fish; steamed green beans; mashed potatoes; whole-grain roll; raspberry sherbet
SATURDAY	Half a grapefruit; two slices whole-grain toast with peanut butter; banana shake made with skim milk	Salad of lettuce, low-fat cottage cheese, peaches, and walnuts; two oat bran muffins with soft margarine	Rice with beans and chopped bell peppers, onions, tomatoes, olives; low-fat rice pudding
SUNDAY	Fresh fruit with low-fat plain yogurt; two-egg omelette; one or two slices whole-grain toast with soft margarine or jelly	Roast chicken with roasted potatoes, carrots, and fennel; whole-grain roll with soft margarine; poached pears	Pasta with tomato-based sauce; spinach and red onion salad; low-fat frozen chocolate yogurt

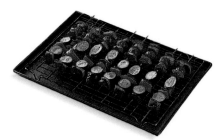

VEGETABLE KEBABS
Skewer cubed peppers, zucchini, and baby tomatoes. Marinate in low-sodium soy sauce, herbs, and spices, as desired; broil until lightly browned on all sides.

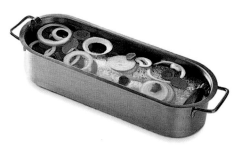

POACHED FISH
Place fish in a poaching pan or large saucepan with sliced carrots, onions, a bay leaf, and other herbs. Cover with water and simmer until fish flakes easily.

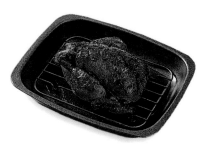

ROAST CHICKEN
Coat chicken with mustard and spices or a little honey. Roast on a rack to allow fat to drain away, covering with foil for the first part of roasting.

COFFEE CONNECTION
Caffeine has no proven connection to heart disease; nevertheless, it should be used in moderation because it constricts blood vessels and can also cause palpitations.

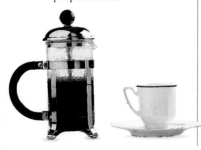

ALCOHOL AND YOUR HEART

Moderate drinkers may have a lower risk of heart disease than people who do not drink at all. In a study of alcohol intake and heart disease risk at Harvard University in 1993, drinking two standard alcoholic drinks every day for six weeks increased the HDL cholesterol in participants by 17 percent. This rise can be interpreted as a 40 percent reduction in the risk of heart disease.

A 1994 study in the Netherlands, led by H. Hendriks, investigated the influence of moderate alcohol intake on the clotting mechanism. The alcohol was imbibed before and during the evening meal in the form of beer, red wine, or gin. The results showed that all forms of alcohol activated reactions that may help blood clots dissolve and prevent new ones from forming.

While health experts acknowledge the protective qualities of moderate alcohol consumption, they are quick to emphasize that this does not mean teetotallers should start drinking. In fact, consuming grapes or grape juice, especially red varieties, seems to provide as many or more bioflavonoids as drinking wine (see below).

How much alcohol is beneficial?

The beneficial effects of alcohol appear to occur with no more than one drink a day for women, two for men. One drink equals a 12-ounce beer, a 4-ounce glass of wine, a 2½-ounce martini, and a 7½-ounce gin and tonic.

Those who have more than one or two daily drinks offset the benefits because high intakes of alcohol tend to increase blood pressure, itself a risk factor for heart disease. Drinking a lot of alcohol, which is relatively high in calories (7 per gram), also tends to cause weight gain, another risk factor for heart disease. Other problems connected with high alcohol intake include liver disease, damage to the kidneys and brain, and an increased risk of low-birth-weight babies and fetal alcohol syndrome.

Why is wine special?

Some studies suggest that wine has a more powerful effect in protecting against heart disease than beer or spirits. Various theories explaining why have been offered. In addition to the properties cited in the studies above, wine, especially red wine, has bioflavonoids that provide antioxidant effects. It is possible, too, that many wine drinkers have

healthier lifestyles than beer and spirit drinkers. Some experts believe the difference is not so much what is in the drink as who is drinking it. In the United States wine drinkers tend to be women, nonsmokers, better educated, and moderate drinkers—all factors associated with a lower risk of heart disease.

IRON OVERLOAD

While the human body needs a steady supply of iron for healthy blood cells to transport oxygen, too much of this mineral can cause irreversible damage to the heart. Even moderately elevated iron levels may set the stage for heart disease. Unfortunately, iron overload does not usually produce symptoms (ruddy skin, chronic fatigue, joint and intestinal pain, irregular heartbeat) until a damaging amount of iron has accumulated in muscle tissue, the liver, bone marrow, spleen, and other organs. (A special blood test can detect iron overload.)

One theory is that excess iron injures artery walls and promotes the formation of fatty deposits. Some researchers believe that the iron in a high-meat diet may promote heart disease even more than a high-fat diet alone.

Genetic factors influence iron absorption; about 10 percent of whites and 30 percent of African Americans carry a gene that predisposes them to store extra iron. Men and postmenopausal women are especially vulnerable. Anyone who is predisposed to conserve iron should avoid foods that are high in iron and supplements of vitamin C, which increases the body's absorption of iron.

CAFFEINE AND YOUR HEART

Studies of a connection between caffeine and high blood pressure and a related increased risk of heart disease are inconclusive. However, doctors still recommend that people with hypertension restrict their intake of caffeine because it increases adrenaline production, which causes blood vessels to constrict. Drinking two to three cups of coffee or cola drinks a day is unlikely to induce problems with your heart, but excessive caffeine may cause palpitations (see page 87), so people who have been diagnosed with arrhythmias should avoid caffeine.

Coffee may raise blood cholesterol levels if boiled for about 10 minutes, the practice in Scandinavia, or made in a French-press coffeepot. Filtered, espresso, and instant coffees do not have this effect.

CHAPTER 4

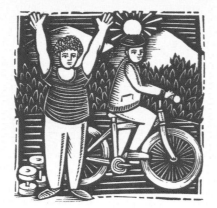

EXERCISING TO PROTECT YOUR HEART

A daily exercise regimen can be extolled simply because it promotes general fitness and well-being. But the benefits of a controlled program extend even further in its effects on the heart. The more regularly you induce the body's pump to work harder, the more you build up a defense against cardiovascular disease. An exercise program can be tailored to any level of fitness but should be planned in consultation with a doctor.

EXERCISE AND YOUR HEART

A regular exercise program can make an important contribution to your well-being. Vigorous physical activity improves the functioning of your heart, lungs, and circulatory system.

Falling heart rate

This graph shows the effect of regular exercise on a middle-aged man's resting heart rate.

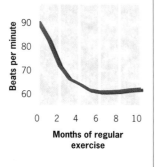

Cardiac output

A fit person uses oxygen more efficiently. As demand on the heart increases, it does not have to pump as much blood per minute to meet oxygen requirements.

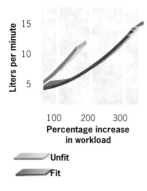

A sedentary lifestyle is among the varied causes of cardiovascular diseases, and with today's labor-saving technology, many people have less need to exert themselves physically. A low level of exercise alone rarely strikes down an otherwise healthy individual, but many studies make it clear that exercise can help in both the prevention of and recovery from heart disease.

Physical fitness plays a central role in many of the programs designed to prevent heart disease. It is now regularly prescribed for people who already suffer heart problems. Patients who have had a heart attack or undergone angioplasty or coronary artery bypass surgery are often encouraged to begin medically supervised exercise regimens within two weeks of leaving the hospital.

THE BENEFITS OF EXERCISE

The short-term benefits of exercise include greater physical and mental energy, relief of stress, and more self-confidence. Regular long-term physical activity can lessen the chance of stroke and coronary artery disease. (A major study of middle-aged women found that walking fast—about three miles per hour—for 30 minutes a day can cut the risk of heart attack by up to 40 percent.) It can also reduce blood pressure and cholesterol levels, prevent osteoporosis, and help maintain a healthy body weight. For exercise to be beneficial in the long term it needs to be done regularly and over an extended period. If you quit after a few months, any benefits you have gained will rapidly disappear.

Exercise and the heart muscle

During exercise muscles require more blood to keep them supplied with oxygen and fuel. The volume of blood entering the heart increases and the heart has to contract more forcefully to eject it. With regular exercise the heart muscle becomes stronger and its blood vessels proliferate (that is, more capillaries grow), thus improving its ability to pump blood and making it more efficient. In fact, this proliferation of blood vessels occurs in all muscles that are worked regularly.

A healthier, fitter heart pumps more blood with each beat and can decrease its work rate while sustaining the same level of flow, resulting in a lower resting pulse. As fitness increases, the exercise pulse rate also slows, and the pulse returns to its resting level more quickly.

Exercise and fat burning

Keeping your weight within recommended limits is important for the health of your heart. Excess weight puts strain on the heart, which has to work harder to supply blood to the extra tissue. Less body fat also means a reduced risk of disease-causing cholesterol accumulating in the arteries.

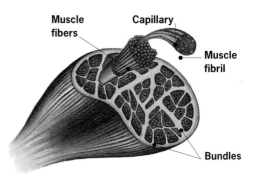

INSIDE A MUSCLE
During exercise the muscle fibers produce energy by using oxygen to burn glucose, which is supplied by the blood. As more blood is required, the number of capillaries increases.

Sustained low- to moderate-intensity exercise, such as walking or swimming for regular periods of at least 20 to 30 minutes a session, uses energy from fat stores. With regular exercise your body becomes more efficient at accessing fat stores, and the fitter you are, the quicker it will burn fat.

High-intensity exercise, such as sprinting in short spurts, uses energy from glycogen stores in the muscles and, although it burns calories, it does not use up your fat.

Exercise also increases the amount of muscle tissue in the body. Because muscle cells, even at rest, have high energy requirements compared to other cells, more muscle means a higher metabolic rate. This means you burn more calories even while resting.

WHAT IS FITNESS?

Fitness is a general term that encompasses an overall standard of strength, flexibility, and endurance. Your body responds to an increase in the amount or intensity of exercise by adapting and maintaining itself in a more ready state, so that you can initiate and maintain an increased pace whenever the need occurs.

The most important type of exercise for the heart is known as cardiovascular, cardiorespiratory, or aerobic exercise. All of these refer to exertion that requires more oxygen usage by your muscles, which makes you breathe harder and your heart beat faster. Exercises for strength and flexibility may be no less vital to the body as a whole, but they are not as directly important to the heart's healthy functioning.

Assessing your fitness

Before you start an exercise program, it is well worth seeking advice from an exercise professional (see page 72). You can also get an exercise screening (from a personal trainer or health club), which looks at your way of life, medical background, and previous exercise patterns in order to assess your aims and needs in a fitness regimen.

Starting with caution

Ideally, an aerobic exercise program should be entered into only after a proper evaluation of any cardiovascular risk factors. These include levels of cholesterol and triglycerides in the blood, blood pressure, family history of premature heart disease, and any chronic illness, such as asthma.

Other types of exercise should be treated with even more caution: strenuous activities, like lifting and holding heavy weights or squeezing muscles tightly for extended periods, may strain the skeleton and the heart and elevate blood pressure to high levels.

If your blood pressure is 140/90 or lower, then you can exercise safely. However, if it is higher than this, you need to speak to your doctor about precautions you should take when exercising and have your blood pressure checked regularly.

Also, you should consult with your doctor if you have recently suffered an illness or have not exercised for a very long time. It is important to feel confident that there will be no hidden problems that might suddenly develop when you begin exercising.

COMPONENTS OF FITNESS

The basic elements of any good physical fitness program are exercises designed to increase endurance, flexibility, and strength. Dynamic, or aerobic, exercise will increase

Exercise really helps

The Framingham (Massachusetts) Heart Study of 5,000 people, which began in 1948 and continued for over 40 years, has confirmed that people who do little or no exercise are at greater risk of heart disease than those who do regular, moderate exercise.

Over a period of 12 years, researchers found that those people who had very low levels of activity were five times more likely to die from heart disease than very active people. In cases of sudden death from heart attack, there was a direct and consistent statistical relation to poor fitness.

HOW EXERCISE AFFECTS YOUR BODY
When you exercise, your body is put under physical stress. The central nervous system and adrenal glands produce the hormones noradrenaline and adrenaline, which cause changes that help your body work as efficiently as possible.

Skin—Blood vessels contract so that more blood can reach the muscles.

Lungs take in more oxygen, needed by the muscles as breathing rate and depth increase.

Heart speeds up to pump a greater volume of blood to active muscles and pumps more blood per beat.

Muscles—Blood vessels dilate so that blood flow is increased, and more oxygen, glycogen, and minerals are supplied to enable muscle contraction.

Digestive system—Blood vessels contract so that more blood can go to the muscles.

The talk test

A simple way to test whether you are exercising to much or too little is to see if during the activity you are able to carry on a conversation. While working at 50 to 60 percent of your maximum heart rate, it should be possible to converse without undue disruption to breathing. At 70 to 80 percent (for most people this is the desirable goal) your conversation will be punctuated by increased breathing. If you are too winded to talk, you are probably overdoing it and should slow down your pace.

endurance and has the most positive effect on the health of the cardiovascular system. High-intensity, or strength exercises, which are often referred to as anaerobic, are important for overall fitness.

Endurance

Aerobic endurance, or stamina, refers to the capacity to postpone fatigue and keep going without gasping for breath or suffering other discomfort. To improve stamina you need to improve the efficiency of your heart and lungs by undertaking regular exercise that lasts for an extended period of time.

Intensity of the exercise is important. You should measure your heart rate before, during, and after exercising, aiming for your target heart-rate zone (see page 70). This goal varies according to fitness level. With regular exercise, as your heart becomes stronger, you can work toward the higher range of your target zone.

Flexibility

Stretching increases the range of movement in the body's joints, improves the elasticity of the muscles that work the joints, tightens and tones the joints themselves, and also

shortens and strengthens the supporting ligaments. Stretching also helps to slow the decline in mobility that comes with aging, relieves tension in tired muscles, and can help reduce overall stress levels. Because stress is a contributing factor in heart problems, stretching is always a useful part of an exercise program, and it balances periods of exertion as well.

Effective stretching is carried out using safe "static" techniques, which involve moving slowly into certain postures and holding them for 10 to 30 seconds. Such movements are an excellent way to start the morning or unwind at the end of a stressful day. Try stretching to soothing music for a very effective relaxation session.

Strength

To make muscles and bones stronger, carefully controlled strength exercises should form part of any exercise routine, even though they do not directly affect the heart. Weight-bearing exercises play an important role in the prevention of osteoporosis (bone weakening disease), but sufferers of coronary artery disease or high blood pressure should approach them carefully.

THE FITNESS COMBINATION

A well-balanced exercise program should include an aerobic, stretching, and toning component to achieve maximum fitness and health. On pages 78 to 81 you will find more exercises for stretching and toning various parts of your body.

Handweights should be very light for toning.

Stretch all main muscle groups.

STRETCHING FOR FLEXIBILITY Stretches before or after exercise sessions should be specific to the muscles that will be used. However, a general stretching session can be done at any time for stress relief.

AEROBIC FOR ENDURANCE Rowing is a good aerobic exercise, as long as it is maintained for at least 20 minutes a session, several times per week.

TONING AND STRENGTH Lightweight strength exercises tone your muscles and make joints and muscles stronger.

Exercise machines provide a good aerobic workout.

Exercises to improve strength and muscle tone can be performed with handheld weights, wrist and/or ankle weights, elastic resistance bands, or machines and should target all the joints and muscles in a balanced way. They must be suited to the individual's fitness level and performed slowly and carefully within a joint's normal range of movement. Such exercises will not make you muscle-bound because the weights used are light and the time period is not sufficient to build up visible muscle tissue.

TEST YOUR FITNESS

Try these three tests to find out how fit you are. Keep a record of your scores and redo the tests after a month of regular exercise. If you are not improving, you are probably not working hard enough. You may wish to seek the advice of a personal trainer (see page 72).

AEROBIC FITNESS INDEX RATING

Calculate your aerobic fitness index (AFI) and compare it with the chart below to see how fit you are.

Poor	0–50
Fair	50–79
Good	80–99
Very good	100–119
Excellent	120+

ENDURANCE STEP TEST
Step up and down in time with a metronome beat or dance music for 5 minutes. Sit down for a minute and take your pulse for 30 seconds. To calculate your aerobic fitness index (AFI), divide 30,000 by your 30-second pulse multiplied by 5.5. For example, if your 30-second pulse is 50, your AFI equals 109 (30,000 divided by 50 x 5.5).

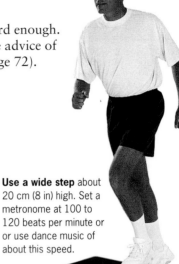

Use a wide step about 20 cm (8 in) high. Set a metronome at 100 to 120 beats per minute or or use dance music of about this speed.

MUSCLE STRENGTH RATING

To score, count how many curl-ups you can do in 1 minute and match them against your age and sex.

AGE	20–35	36–50	51–70
WOMEN			
Poor	45	35	25
Fair	50	40	30
Good	55	45	35
Very good	60	50	40
Excellent	65+	55+	45+
MEN			
Poor	50	40	30
Fair	55	45	35
Good	60	50	40
Very good	65	55	45
Excellent	75+	65+	55+

STRENGTH CURL-UP TEST
Lie on your back, knees bent, feet flat on the floor. Keep your lower back pressed against the floor at all times. Place your hands on top of your thighs. Curl your shoulders forward off the floor and slide your hands up along your legs toward your kneecaps. Uncurl. Repeat for 1 minute.

FLEXIBILITY RATING

To score, see where your fingers touch the tape and match the distance against your age and sex.

Try to keep your back straight as you reach forward.

FLEXIBILITY SIT AND REACH TEST
Lay a tape measure on the floor and secure it to the floor with tape at the 30 cm (12 in) mark and the 75 cm (30 in) mark. Sit astride the tape at the zero mark with legs outstretched and slightly apart.

Slowly reach forward with both hands toward your heels. Hold for 3 seconds.

AGE	20–35	36–50	51–70
WOMEN	CM (IN)	CM (IN)	CM (IN)
Poor	40 (15)	35 (14)	30 (12)
Fair	50 (20)	45 (18)	40 (15)
Good	60 (24)	55 (22)	50 (20)
Very good	70 (28)	65 (26)	60 (24)
Excellent	80 (32)	75 (30)	65 (26)
MEN			
Poor	30 (12)	25 (10)	20 (8)
Fair	40 (15)	35 (14)	30 (12)
Good	50 (20)	45 (18)	40 (15)
Very good	60 (24)	55 (22)	50 (20)
Excellent	65 (26)	60 (24)	55 (22)

Blood pressure and fitness

Regular exercise can help reduce high blood pressure. However, if your blood pressure is very high, you will have to avoid certain kinds of strenuous exercise, such as weight lifting.

You should have your blood pressure checked by your doctor. If it is 140/90 or lower, then you can exercise safely. However, if it is higher than this, ask your doctor to advise you about a safe exercise program and have your blood pressure checked regularly.

MONITORING YOUR FITNESS

Most people are completely unaware of how fit their heart really is. Yet it pays to find out so you can work safely toward certain targets that will keep your heart healthy. There are a number of basic self-assessment tests.

You can find out what your maximum heart rate potential and target heart rate zone should be by checking the chart at right. Then perform the tests shown on page 69 to get an idea of your endurance, flexibility, and strength—the three major components of fitness. If you have not exercised for a long time, do these tests with caution, taking each stage gradually, and be sure to stop immediately if you feel some discomfort. In order to monitor your progress, repeat the tests every few weeks after beginning your exercise program. Be sure to warm up properly before starting any exercise (see page 78).

Rate of perceived exertion

A simple way to check that you are exercising at the right intensity is to assess how you feel while doing it. The rate of perceived exertion (RPE) is a very quick yet surprisingly accurate way of monitoring your exercise intensity (see table below). It works on the assumption that if you perceive you are working hard, then you probably are, and your heart rate is likely to be in the target zone. The scale runs from 6 (no exertion) to 20 (maximum exertion). By adding a zero to each number, you can get a rough approximation of your heart rate. For example, at a rate of perceived exertion of 13 (somewhat hard) your heart rate is approximately 130 beats per minute.

PERCEIVED EXERTION RATES

EXERTION LEVEL	RATING
No exertion at all	6
Very very light	7–8
Very light	9–10
Fairly light	11–12
Somewhat hard	13–14
Hard	15–16
Very hard	17–18
Very very hard	19
The limit of exertion	20

TARGET HEART RATE ZONE

Your target heart rate zone (THRZ) is 60 to 90 percent of your maximum heart rate potential and is the range in which fit people should exercise. Unfit people should start at 50 to 60 percent and increase their exertion over a few weeks. To check your THRZ, take your pulse halfway into your exercise session or use a heart rate monitor (see page 97).

AGE	MAXIMUM HEART RATE	60% LEVEL	90% LEVEL
20	200	120	180
25	195	117	175
30	190	114	171
35	185	111	167
40	180	108	162
45	175	105	158
50	170	102	153
55	165	99	149
60	160	96	144
65	155	93	140
70	150	90	135

Maximum heart rate

Any exertion that makes your heart beat faster is good for it. To get the most from exercise, however, you need to perform at a rate that is sufficiently difficult to give your heart a thorough workout but not so difficult that you are forced to stop after only a few minutes.

The maximum heart rate potential (MHR) is the uppermost level at which your heart can beat during exertion; it varies according to age. The formula for the calculation is 220 minus your age. So a 40-year-old person will have an MHR of 180. However, you should not aim to exercise at your MHR because you will not be able to sustain this level of intensity, and it is not healthy for your heart. Once you know your MHR, you can calculate your target heart rate zone (see above) and make your heart work comfortably within it.

According to the scale above, a 40-year-old person of average fitness should aim to exercise at a heart rate of 108 to 162 beats per minute. A very unfit person should aim to exercise at 50 to 60 percent of his or her MHR and build up gradually to 90 percent.

AEROBIC EXERCISE
Riding at moderate speed for at least 20 minutes burns extra calories and is good for your heart.

AEROBIC AND ANAEROBIC EXERCISE

Aerobic exercise is any prolonged activity, done for at least 20 minutes, that increases the heart rate and uses oxygen to produce energy for the muscles. It includes walking, jogging, bicycling, skiing, aerobic dancing, swimming, such racquet sports as tennis and squash, and team sports like basketball.

Anaerobic exercise refers to short, sharp bursts of strenuous activity in which the oxygen supply in the blood stream is not sufficient to provide energy quickly enough to the muscles, so the muscles use a chemical process without oxygen to break down carbohydrates. Sprinting and weight lifting are anaerobic exercises.

The benefits of aerobic exercise

Even a slight increase in the intensity of exertion will require the heart to perform more work to pump blood around the body and keep pace with the muscles' demand for oxygenated blood. Exercise of low to moderate intensity allows the heart to increase its workload gradually and thus enables it to work longer at a steady pace. This is far better for your heart and muscles than short bursts of strenuous exercise.

Aerobic exercise of low to moderate intensity is the key to a healthy heart and circulatory system. With regular aerobic exercise the heart, lungs, and blood vessels are all called upon to work hard more frequently, and they become ever more efficient and perform their tasks with less stress. So exercise that felt difficult to begin with gradually becomes much easier.

For the full benefits of aerobic exercise you may wish to join a gym. Most offer a wide variety of classes that vary in intensity and level of difficulty. Step classes, for example, involve a routine of exercises done stepping up and down on a box. When you join a gym you should get a fitness assessment and be advised as to which class level you should start with. Later, you should be told when you are ready to move up a level.

EFFECTIVE EXERCISE

The degree of pleasure that you get from exercising is likely to determine how long you stick to it and thus its effectiveness. It is important, therefore, to choose your exercises carefully. A key question is whether you want to exercise alone or in a group. For some, exercising alone is more attractive because of the privacy, relaxing solitude, and convenience it provides. The activity and location can be tailored to an individual's schedule. Other people prefer the social interaction and mutual encouragement that a group activity offers. Exercising with a friend affords not only companionship but also motivation.

What about sports?

Another important factor in choosing activities is what you want to achieve with the exercise. While aerobic dancing can play an important role in helping you become and stay healthy, an activity such as weight lifting may not. And team sports like football, basketball, and baseball are better for people who are already in good shape than those who aren't. In particular, a sport like squash, which demands a high intensity of activity, requires a good deal of physical preparation if it is to exercise the heart safely and effectively.

Sporadic involvement in a high-intensity exercise or sport, such as a game of football or basketball, can overstrain an unfit heart. A sound low-to-moderate aerobic exercise program, supported by regular work on strength and flexibility, is more effective in restoring or maintaining basic fitness than any strenuous participation in sports. It is wise to bear in mind the motto, "Get fit to play sports, don't play sports to get fit."

AEROBIC EXERCISE FACTS

Aerobic exercise always has the same features.

▶ *It lasts for at least 20 minutes per session.*

▶ *Its intensity is low to moderate.*

▶ *It can be sustained over a long period of time.*

▶ *It uses oxygen for energy-creating processes.*

▶ *It improves the cardiovascular system.*

▶ *It improves fitness.*

ANAEROBIC EXERCISE
Because squash involves short spurts of very intense activity, a person must already be fairly fit before undertaking this sport.

The Personal Trainer

If you are particularly concerned about improving the health of your heart, a personal trainer can devise a program with that aim in mind. More and more people are enlisting a trainer's special skills when they embark on fitness regimens.

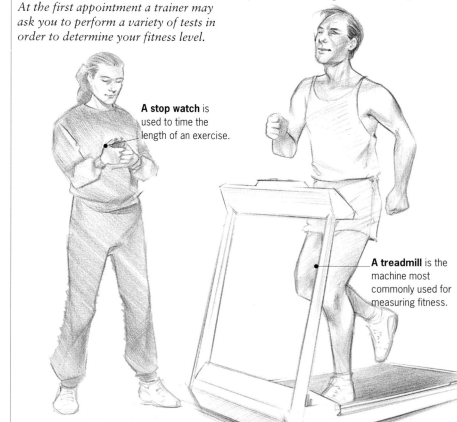

WHAT TO WEAR
Buy the appropriate shoes for your chosen type of exercise. They should be supportive and well-cushioned. Wear comfortable clothing that allows you to move freely and absorbs perspiration. Cotton fabrics are usually best for this, although some people prefer the newer synthetics that wick perspiration away from the body. Dress in layers for cold weather.

ASSESSING YOUR FITNESS
At the first appointment a trainer may ask you to perform a variety of tests in order to determine your fitness level.

A stop watch is used to time the length of an exercise.

A treadmill is the machine most commonly used for measuring fitness.

Personal trainers use their expert knowledge of fitness to devise and conduct exercise programs that are tailored to an individual's special needs and level of fitness.

In the United States many personal trainers have a degree or diploma in sports science or exercise studies. Most have also completed special courses and have a personal trainer's certificate in addition to the basic qualifications. A trainer should carry professional insurance and be certified in cardiopulmonary resuscitation (CPR) and first aid. To check your trainer's qualifications, contact the American Council on Exercise (ACE) in San Diego, California.

A trainer who is registered with the Canadian Alliance of Professional Personal Fitness Trainers has a degree in exercise sciences/human movement plus two to five years of fitness, exercise, and rehabilitation work and CPR training.

Why should I use a personal trainer?
A personal trainer is truly helpful if you need individual attention to improve your technique and could use some extra motivation. He or she can not only design a fitness program for you but also adapt it regularly to suit your circumstances and preferences and make it fun.

Having a personal trainer means that you can arrange sessions when you find it most convenient, at a time and place that suits you—first thing in the morning, for example, at home or in the office or a health club.

In addition to giving you advice on exercise, he or she should be able to suggest a suitable diet and advise you on the management of stress, all of which are essential for a healthy heart. Most important, the trainer can keep you constantly motivated to stay with your program and at the same time make sure that you use good, safe techniques to avoid injury and derive the greatest benefit.

What happens at the first consultation?
Your trainer will discuss your health, fitness goals, and lifestyle and have you fill out a health questionnaire

that covers your medical history, including any incidence of heart disease, high blood pressure, or back problems. This information is then used by your trainer to create a suitable program for you. Together you will decide how many weeks you wish to commit to and how you will achieve your goals. This first meeting also allows you and your trainer to get to know each other.

Will I need to take any tests?

This depends upon your aims. If your purpose is to lose weight, then your trainer may just take some basic measurements, such as your height, weight, and body fat percentage (by measuring the thickness of a pinch of fat on your upper arm against the circumference of your arm). This information will be used as a yardstick to measure your progress. If your aim is to improve and monitor your fitness, he or she may decide to carry out a more detailed fitness assessment to check your endurance, flexibility, and strength.

How much will it cost?

Personal trainers' fees can vary enormously, depending on where you live, whether you train at home or in a gym, and the reputation of the trainer. Although the cost is moderately high, people who go this route usually feel that the money is well spent because of the improvements in their health. You can ask a local health club for an indication of typical fees and also request a recommendation if you need one.

How often do I need to see a personal trainer?

To achieve your goals and maintain your motivation, you should have regular contact with your trainer. In your first consultation you will probably make an agreement to meet once, twice, or perhaps three times a week. How often you choose to meet will depend on the time you have available and also on what you can afford. Once a week is the minimum, in which case the trainer will also

probably advise you to exercise on your own at least two more times a week. Whatever you decide, you should be exercising a total of at least three times a week.

How many weeks must I commit to initially?

Most trainers will ask you to commit to 10 sessions to start. This could be spread out over 3 to 10 weeks, depending on how often you see the trainer. It is important to undertake this commitment so that you can see results. After this initial period, most trainers would prefer a definite arrangement going forward, but some may be happy to see you for occasional sessions thereafter.

How soon will I see results?

Most beginners should see results within six weeks, perhaps sooner if they exercise more than three times a week. Missing out on any sessions or training sporadically will bring about improvements much more

slowly. Your trainer will monitor your progress and change your program as necessary. If your rate of improvement slows, the trainer may increase the frequency or duration of sessions or raise their intensity.

What if I want to discontinue my personal training program?

It is rare for people to discontinue their program altogether, but there can be extenuating circumstances. Because of work obligations, for example, it may be necessary to reduce the frequency of training sessions. Nevertheless, your trainer should be able to keep you motivated and make sure that you maintain your fitness level, even if you have less time available. Once you have embarked on your program, you must complete the number of sessions you agreed to. Of course, if you are not happy with your trainer for any reason, you may wish to change to a new trainer after this time or continue your training alone.

WHAT YOU CAN DO AT HOME

For motivation and encouragement, consider teaming up with a friend and acting as a personal trainer for each other, or be your own trainer. If you have any heart or other health problems, be sure to consult your doctor first and have regular check-ups. To get started, do the following:

▶ *Write down your long-term fitness goals, then divide these into a series of short-term attainable goals.*

▶ *List the benefits that will help keep you motivated.*

▶ *Think of solutions to any problems you have fitting exercise into your life.*

▶ *Create an exercise plan, listing activities either on a day-by-day or week-by-week basis.*

▶ *Keep an exercise diary, writing down exactly which exercise and how much of it you did and your improvement in fitness levels at each session.*

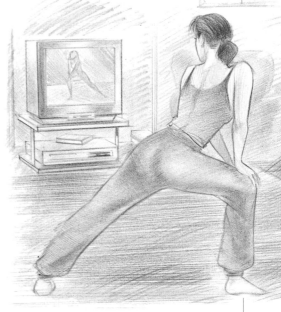

EXERCISING ON YOUR OWN
Videotaped routines are useful for motivation and learning different exercises and the correct way to do them. Set aside specific times for using a tape and ask your family not to disturb you.

MAKING EXERCISE PART OF YOUR LIFE

You may dislike exercise or think you are just too busy for it, but developing an interesting regimen that fits your schedule is not too difficult once you know all the options.

If you want to have or maintain a healthy heart, exercise should be a natural part of your weekly routine. Aerobic exercises (see page 71) are especially beneficial, and a range of activities will provide the most enduring benefits. It will also help you avoid boredom. For instance, you could walk three times per week, swim on Monday, bicycle on Wednesday, and take an aerobics class on Friday. Not only will you exercise all muscle groups without overstraining certain muscles and joints with repetitive movements, but you will find the variety stimulating. When you feel like a rest, just do a stretching routine (see page 78).

CHANGING HABITS

Adding new layers to your routine or altering the familiar pattern of your day rarely comes easily. If you have not exercised for a long time and are quite unfit, you could start off with a daily short exercise, lasting up to five minutes, and build up to the recommended time step by step.

Even when exercise is done for just a short period, the benefits to health are almost immediate. Previously sedentary people embarking on an exercise program for the first time will achieve impressive improvements in aerobic fitness by exercising at very modest intensities of around 50 percent

A FITNESS AND WEIGHT-LOSS PROGRAM

Any fitness regimen aims to improve cardiovascular health, achieve and maintain a healthy weight, and enhance overall well-being. You can use the one below as a guide, but check it first with your doctor. "Aerobics" here refers to classes; as an alternative, you could do circuit training at home (see opposite).

MONDAY	TUESDAY	WEDNESDAY	THURSDAY	FRIDAY	SATURDAY	SUNDAY
WEEK ONE						
Walk 10 min.	Rest	Cycle 10 min.	Rest	Walk 10 min.	Rest	Rest
WEEK TWO						
Cycle 15 min.	Rest	Walk 15 min.	Rest	Swim 15 min.	Rest	Rest
WEEK THREE						
Rest	Walk 25 min.	Rest	Step 45 min.	Rest	Cycle 25 min.	Rest
WEEK FOUR						
Walk 20 min.	Rest	Aerobics 45 min.	Rest	Cycle 20 min.	Rest	Swim 20 min.
WEEK FIVE						
Swim 25 min.	Rest	Step 45 min.	Rest	Walk 25 min.	Rest	Cycle 25 min.
WEEK SIX						
Walk 30 min.	Swim 30 min.	Rest	Aerobics 45 min.	Cycle 30 min.	Rest	Walk 30 min.

CIRCUIT TRAINING

Performing activities in rotation—as shown below—is ideal for cardiovascular fitness and for strengthening different muscle groups. You can join a circuit class at a gym or set up your own circuit at home. Your workout should use different muscle groups and include an aerobic component. Spend 30 seconds to 1 minute on each exercise; keep repeating the circuit for at least 20 minutes.

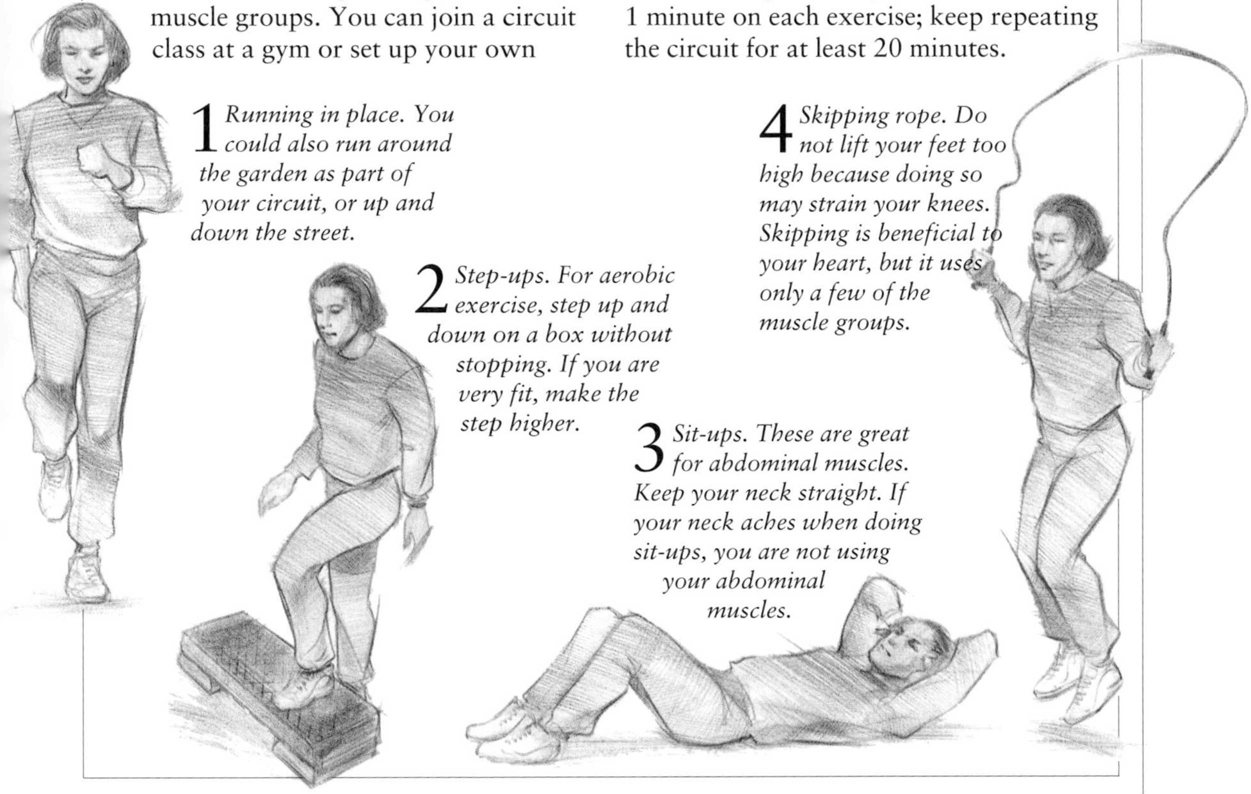

1 Running in place. You could also run around the garden as part of your circuit, or up and down the street.

2 Step-ups. For aerobic exercise, step up and down on a box without stopping. If you are very fit, make the step higher.

3 Sit-ups. These are great for abdominal muscles. Keep your neck straight. If your neck aches when doing sit-ups, you are not using your abdominal muscles.

4 Skipping rope. Do not lift your feet too high because doing so may strain your knees. Skipping is beneficial to your heart, but it uses only a few of the muscle groups.

of maximum heart rate. Sedentary individuals can increase their aerobic capacity by up to 20 percent over an 8-week period by walking or jogging 20 to 30 minutes three times a week at 50 percent of their maximum heart rate.

For people who have made improvements with regular exercise but have then noticed that the rate of improvement is slowing down, an extra stimulus is required to take them further. This can be achieved by making the exercise more intensive or by increasing its duration.

YOUR EXERCISE PROGRAM

A cardiovascular exercise session should start with a 5-minute warm-up, followed by stretching, aerobic exercise for at least 20 minutes, and then a cool-down session.

Warming up

It is essential to warm up before exercising to protect muscles, tendons, and ligaments. March briskly in place or up and down in a small area. Circle hands and feet in both directions to warm up the joints, making them more mobile. Gently stretch muscles that are going to be used in the activity to follow. In cycling, for example, the ankles and hips need special attention; in swimming, it's the shoulders, ankles, and hips. (See page 78 for stretching exercises.) This should take up about five minutes, and your body should feel warm afterward. Start your chosen exercise slowly and then gradually increase the pace.

Cooling down

A cool-down period of about 10 minutes should be included in the schedule. It follows the most intense part of an exercise session, which should last a minimum of 20 minutes, and allows the heart rate to return to normal and sweating to subside. It also prevents muscle cramps and stiffness.

Gradually slow the pace of your exercise, then walk around for a few minutes until your breathing is normal. To slow your breathing, inhale deeply as you raise your arms above your head and exhale as you

IF YOU HAVE A HEART CONDITION

People with diagnosed heart disease should follow these rules.

▶ *Get your doctor's approval to exercise.*

▶ *Start your exercise program at a slow pace and build up gradually.*

▶ *Do not exercise outdoors in extreme weather.*

▶ *Do not do any strenuous exercises.*

▶ *Do not exercise for at least 2 hours after having a bath or eating a meal.*

▶ *Stop exercising immediately if you feel dizzy or faint or experience chest pain, nausea, severe breathlessness, severe palpitations, fatigue, or intense pain.*

AN EXERCISE SESSION

ACTIVITY	MINUTES
Warm up	5
Stretching	5
Aerobic activity	20–30
Cool down	10
Total session	40–50

bring them down next to your sides. Repeat the exercises and stretches that you did in your warm up, paying particular attention to the muscles you have used the most.

Pace yourself

If you are considering embarking on an exercise program without the supervision of a fitness instructor, begin slowly. Even the most gentle exercise can cause some muscle damage if you are unaccustomed to it, and it can make you very sore in the days to follow. If you have not exercised for three to six months, do not feel bad if you cannot do much at first. Even a 20-minute walk three times a week will benefit your heart.

You can try the Fitness and Weight-Loss Program on page 74, but remember that this is intended as a guide only. Remain flexible in your approach and be prepared to adapt and modify the program according to specific situations in your daily life and the kind of aerobic exercise you prefer. If your schedule is too rigid, it may dampen your motivation. More important, you should not exercise if you are injured or ill, although if you have only a mild cold, exercise may be of benefit.

Vary your choice of exercise to help reduce the repetitive strain in joints that may occur when just one activity is practiced. No single aerobic exercise is superior to any other for improving the health of the cardiovascular system.

Always try to exercise at a minimum of 50 to 60 percent of your maximum heart rate (MHR, see page 68). If you have been exercising regularly for at least six months, you may strive to exercise at 60 to 70 percent of your MHR. And if you are in very good shape, aim for 80 to 90 percent.

On days when no aerobic exercise is specified, you don't have the time to fit an aerobic exercise into your schedule, or you are feeling very tired, you could do a stretching or toning routine instead (see pages 78–81) or simply practice some relaxation exercises (see page 82).

EXERCISE EQUIPMENT FOR THE HOME

Exercising at home can be as fun and varied as going to a gym or health club and perhaps more comfortable. The equipment below will ensure that you get a good cardiovascular workout. Always read the instructions for the machine and exercise with caution. Place your exercise machine where you will be certain to use it.

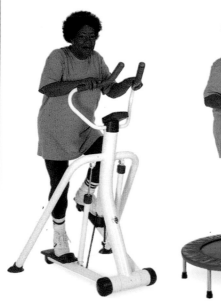

STEP MACHINE
This works the legs and buttocks and gives your heart a workout.

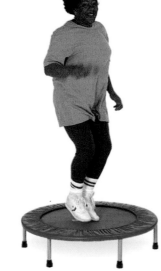

TRAMPOLINE
The most portable of home equipment items, this provides many aerobic benefits.

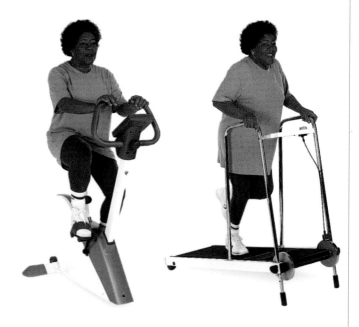

EXERCISE BICYCLE
Bicycles are great for heart and lung fitness, thigh muscle toning, and fat burning.

TREADMILL
With a treadmill you can go for a walk or run, regardless of weather conditions.

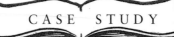

CASE STUDY

An Angina Sufferer

Angina patients often think they cannot exercise without provoking an attack. However, regular exercise of the right kind and intensity can actually make the heart fitter, reduce the number of pain episodes, and improve general health. Undertaking more exercise is one of several lifestyle changes that angina sufferers can make to improve their condition.

Greg is a 51-year-old bank manager married to Sue, a teacher. They have two children. Greg's lifestyle does not lend itself to keeping fit; he has working lunches in restaurants almost every day. Partly because of all the rich food, his weight has crept up over the past five years. At work there have been rumors of branch mergers and redundancies of senior staff, which has caused Greg to incur frequent tension headaches. He has also been feeling uncomfortably breathless after climbing stairs, and he has a tight feeling around his upper chest after walking a short distance. Anxious about his health because his father died from a heart attack in his sixties, he visits his doctor, who diagnoses angina.

WHAT SHOULD GREG DO?

Greg's doctor has prescribed some medication for him to take during his attacks, but Greg must also act to reduce all the factors that are contributing to his angina.

Greg has a moderately raised blood cholesterol level, so he needs to follow a low-fat, balanced diet, as well as to lose some weight. It will be necessary for him to exercise more to aid in weight loss, prevent high blood pressure, and improve his cardiovascular health in general. Getting his family's support in these endeavors will be vital.

Greg should also find ways to reduce his stress levels and increase the amount of time he spends relaxing. Like it or not, he must realistically assess his work future as well.

Action Plan

EXERCISE
Establish a weekly program—some activities by himself, some with Sue and the kids. Possibly join a health club.

STRESS
Talk to area manager about fears for the future. Think about options if the news is not good. Increase relaxation time.

DIET
Check out low-fat and low-calorie options at local restaurants. Cut down on alcohol consumption. Have cholesterol levels checked in three months.

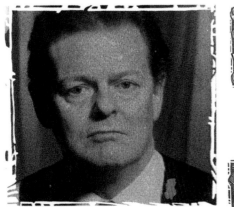

STRESS
Tension and anxiety increases a person's heart rate and can precipitate an attack of angina.

EXERCISE
Physical exertion can mitigate angina because it improves heart rate, blood pressure, volume of blood per heartbeat, and oxygen supply to the heart.

DIET
Being overweight increases the risk of heart disease. A low-fat diet is essential for a healthy heart.

HOW THINGS TURNED OUT FOR GREG

Greg bought bicycles for the family, and they cycle together on weekends. He and Sue go swimming every week. A talk with his manager has reassured him that his job is not presently at risk. This knowledge has reduced his stress levels considerably. He has also taken courses to improve his management techniques. Greg has lost 6.4 kg (14 lb) in three months, his overall cholesterol level is lower, and he has had only one angina attack.

Improving Your Flexibility with

Stretching

Before undertaking any aerobic or strengthening exercise and after all exercise sessions, muscles must be stretched to avoid injury. Stretching is also beneficial for improving flexibility, easing stiffness, reducing stress, and promoting relaxation.

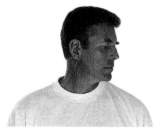

NECK ROTATION
Start your routine with a neck stretch. Begin with your chin on your chest. Roll your head to the right, taking the chin to your right shoulder, then rotate to the left, taking the chin to your left shoulder. Do not roll your head backward.

Before exercising, warm up your body by walking briskly around the block or a room, taking long strides and swinging your arms. Alternatively, you can march in place, lifting your knees and pumping your arms.

Next, stretch out muscles, moving into each position in a slow and controlled way. Do not force yourself or bounce or jerk. Go as far as you comfortably can; the stretches should not feel painful. Learn to relax into each position and breathe normally.

Perform the complete routine twice. As you become more flexible, hold the stretches for a few seconds longer, eventually building up to 30 seconds for each one.

STRETCHES FOR THE UPPER BODY

Make sure you feel warm and relaxed. Start with feet shoulder width apart and back straight. Keep knees and elbows flexible, not rigid.

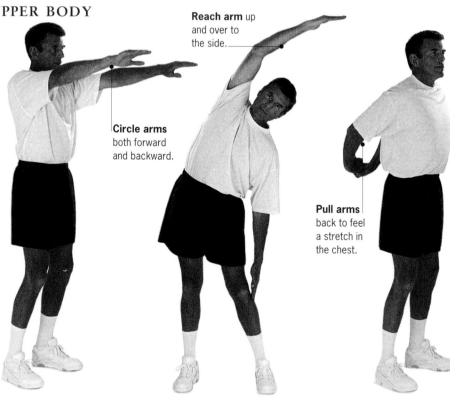

Clasp fingers
with palms facing downward.

Reach arm up and over to the side.

Circle arms
both forward and backward.

Pull arms
back to feel a stretch in the chest.

UPPER BACK
Bend knees slightly. Raise both arms above your head and as you breathe in, interlock fingers and stretch arms upward as far as possible. Hold for 10 seconds, then exhale as you release.

SHOULDER CIRCLES
Raise your arms straight up in front of you. Move your arms slowly backward six times, then forward six times, making circles.

WAIST STRETCH
Reach up with your right arm and then bend to your left, placing your other hand on the side of your thigh. Hold for 10 seconds, then repeat on the other side.

CHEST STRETCH
Clasp your hands behind your back, elbows slightly bent, and pull your shoulders back and toward each other. Hold for 10 seconds.

78

STRETCHES FOR THE LOWER BODY

Muscle strain is most common in the legs, so stretching leg muscles is essential before and after jogging, cycling, skiing, dancing, tennis, squash, and field sports. Gentle stretching of the lower back is also important before and after exercise, but should be done with caution.

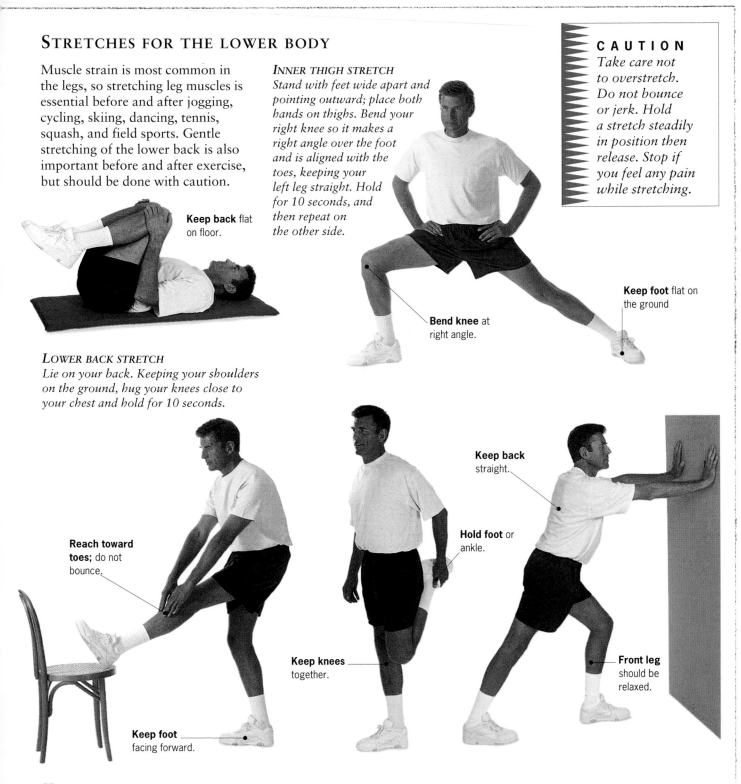

Keep back flat on floor.

INNER THIGH STRETCH
Stand with feet wide apart and pointing outward; place both hands on thighs. Bend your right knee so it makes a right angle over the foot and is aligned with the toes, keeping your left leg straight. Hold for 10 seconds, and then repeat on the other side.

Bend knee at right angle.

Keep foot flat on the ground

LOWER BACK STRETCH
Lie on your back. Keeping your shoulders on the ground, hug your knees close to your chest and hold for 10 seconds.

Reach toward toes; do not bounce.

Keep back straight.

Hold foot or ankle.

Keep knees together.

Front leg should be relaxed.

Keep foot facing forward.

HAMSTRING STRETCH
Place right heel on a chair. Keeping leg straight, bend toward the leg until you feel a stretch in your hamstrings (at the back of the thigh). Hold for 6 to 10 seconds and then repeat with the other leg.

FRONT THIGH STRETCH
Standing with feet together, bend your left leg back and hold on to your ankle or foot, keeping thighs parallel. Hold for 6 to 10 seconds and then repeat with the other leg.

CALF STRETCH
Place both hands on a wall at shoulder height, arms straight. Move your feet back until your legs are at a 45-degree angle to the floor. Bring left foot forward, keeping right leg straight. Adjust distance between feet until you feel a stretch in your right calf. Hold for 6 to 10 seconds and then repeat with other leg.

Toning

An exercise regimen needs to include a toning component, as well as stretching and cardiovascular activities. A toning program firms your muscles, strengthens your body, and improves your overall shape and posture.

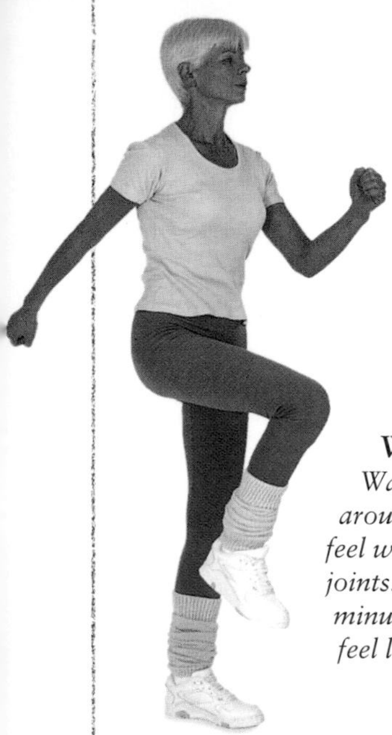

WARMING UP
Walk briskly in place or around the room until you feel warm. Rotate your joints. Stretch for 15 minutes until the muscles feel loosened.

Even if toning does not contribute directly to cardiovascular health, increased muscle means a higher metabolic rate and more efficient burning of energy in your body.

If you have high blood pressure or a diagnosed heart condition, you should consult your doctor before

doing these exercises. Always warm up before toning to avoid injury.

Hand weights are used in some of the exercises shown below. Choose very light ones to start (1 kg/2 lb); you can move to heavier ones as fitness improves, but remember, the aim is to tone, not build muscle bulk.

TONING EXERCISES FOR THE LEGS

Always keep your back straight when doing these exercises. Do only as much as you feel comfortable with. Stop if you feel very tired.

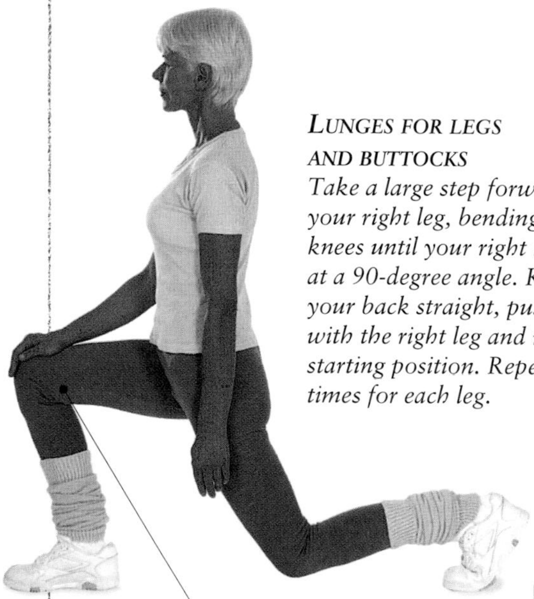

Shoulders should be relaxed.

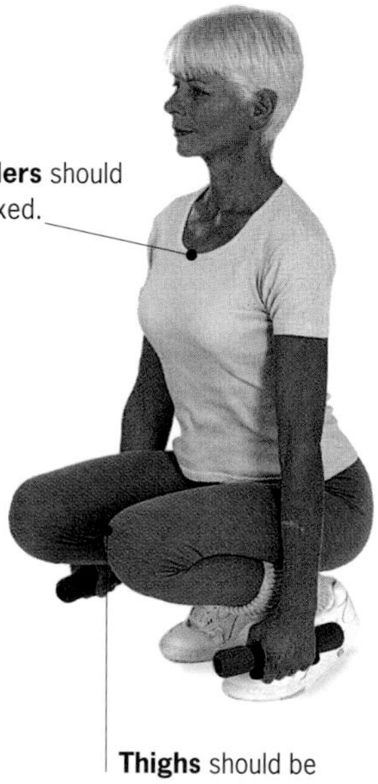

SQUATS FOR LEGS
AND BUTTOCKS
Stand with feet just over shoulder-width apart and hold hand weights in each hand. Squat down, keeping knees in line with toes. Return to starting position. Repeat 20 times.

LUNGES FOR LEGS
AND BUTTOCKS
Take a large step forward with your right leg, bending both knees until your right knee is at a 90-degree angle. Keeping your back straight, push back with the right leg and return to starting position. Repeat 10 times for each leg.

Thighs should be parallel to floor and back should be erect.

TIPS FOR TONING

Hand weights are optional. They should always be light enough to do at least 10 repetitions without causing muscle strain. When your strength improves, you can increase the number of repetitions or use heavier weights. But it is more important to do each exercise correctly than to strain to increase repetitions or weight.

Always breathe out as you move into the exercise, and breathe in as you relax out of it.

Do not use hand weights if you have been diagnosed with high blood pressure.

Knee should be over ankle

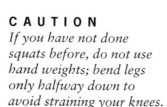

CAUTION
If you have not done squats before, do not use hand weights; bend legs only halfway down to avoid straining your knees.

UPPER BODY TONING

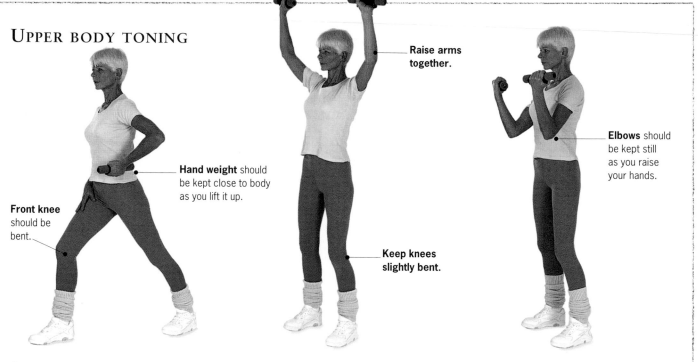

Raise arms together.

Hand weight should be kept close to body as you lift it up.

Front knee should be bent.

Keep knees slightly bent.

Elbows should be kept still as you raise your hands.

ONE-ARM ROWS FOR UPPER BACK
Hold weight in left hand. Step forward with right foot. Start with left arm hanging down, then pull weight up toward waist, bending at elbow. Slowly lower. Repeat 20 times with each arm.

SHOULDER PRESS
Stand straight with feet facing forward. Hold hand weights at shoulder level, palms facing forward. Straighten arms as you push the weights upward, then slowly lower them. Repeat 20 times.

BICEP CURLS
Hold hand weights by your sides. Slowly curl up the weights, bringing hands toward your shoulders. Keep your upper arms still. Return to starting position. Repeat 20 times.

Keep back flat.

PRESS-UPS FOR CHEST AND TRICEPS
Start on all fours. Place hands apart just beyond shoulder width. Slowly lower upper body until elbows are bent at a 90-degree angle, but do not rest on the floor. Push yourself up using your arms. Keep abdomen taut. Repeat 20 times.

BENCH DIPS FOR TRICEPS
Sit on the edge of a sturdy chair, hands beside you, fingers facing forward. Keep feet flat on the floor and knees bent. Move your buttocks forward just free of the chair and lower yourself, bending your elbows to a 90-degree angle and taking your body weight on your arms. Straighten your arms back to starting position. Repeat 20 times.

ABDOMINAL TONING

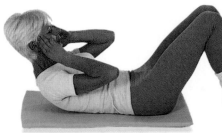

CURL-UPS FOR ABDOMINAL MUSCLES
Lie on your back, knees bent, feet flat on floor. Place hands on your temples. Curl your head and shoulders off the floor as you breathe out, hold for 1 to 2 seconds, then slowly uncurl. Keep lower back on the floor at all times. Repeat 20 times.

COOL DOWN
Stretch all the main muscle groups (see page 78) and walk around slowly until your body has cooled down.

THE ART OF RELAXATION

Relaxation exercises can help relieve stress, thereby reducing your risk of high blood pressure and heart problems, as well as improving your quality of life.

A quick relaxation technique

Lie down on a carpeted floor or on a blanket or pad laid on a bare floor. Starting with the toes, tense each set of muscles as you breathe in. Hold for two seconds at maximum tension, then release gradually as you breathe out. Using the same technique, move up to the ankles, calves, knees, thighs, and so on—even your scalp and ears can hold tension. Try to avoid doing the routine with a scowl of concentration on your face. Repeat the exercise two or three times to promote relaxation and increase circulation to tense areas.

Anxiety often manifests itself as headaches, knitted brows, aching neck and shoulder muscles, and back pains. The Framingham (Massachusetts) Heart Study, which examined risk factors in 5,000 people, monitored the psychological profiles of more than 1,000 volunteers over a period of 40 years. The results suggest that stress does not stop at causing minor aches and pains but can precipitate hypertension, or high blood pressure, the long-term and less tangible effects of which may have life-threatening implications.

The mechanism is still unclear. However, it is known that stress and tension raise the level of adrenaline in the blood, which in turn causes blood vessels to contract and forces the heart to pump harder, thereby raising blood pressure. In addition, higher adrenaline levels may raise cholesterol levels. Stress is therefore associated with an increased chance of heart disease because prolonged hypertension and raised cholesterol are major factors in coronary heart disease.

RELAXATION
Find a quiet place to lie down. Your back should be flat, but you can raise your head slightly on a pillow if you choose. Make sure you are not too warm or too cold, and that no one will disturb you.

COMBATING DISEASE WITH RELAXATION

Recent studies conducted in the United States show that relaxation is one of the most important safeguards against hypertension and heart disease. Another study, by C. Patel back in 1981, reported in the *British Medical Journal*, showed that heart patients who were trained in relaxation techniques stayed healthier for considerably longer periods than untrained patients on hypertensive medication. Whether for prevention or as a cure, following a regular relaxation program is therefore a sound step in promoting the health of the heart.

In addition to fighting stress and hypertension, the power of the mind can be used to ward off other illnesses. In 1991 Dr. Karen Olness, a professor of pediatrics at Case Western Reserve University in Ohio, taught a group of hemophiliacs a way to reduce bleeding after an injury. By using relaxation techniques, they were able to lower their blood pressure and slow blood loss. Some members of the group also used visualization (see page 83) to control their bleeding. One child in the group imagined tiny airplanes flying through his veins, dropping clotting bombs to stop the bleeding.

Despite such promising findings, some doctors are still not convinced that relaxation and visualizsation can really help control disease. Relaxation exercises, however, have certainly been found to ease the physical discomforts of minor illnesses, which drain energy, and creative visualization exercises may help in fighting illnesses caused by stress, including heart disease.

Some people do not believe that they have much imagination and expect visualization to be difficult. In fact, everyone uses their

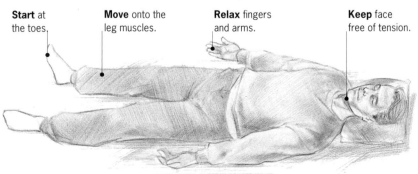

Start at the toes.

Move onto the leg muscles.

Relax fingers and arms.

Keep face free of tension.

mental abilities to create images all the time. If you are asked to think of how to get to the supermarket, your imagination will make a series of pictures showing you the way. If you are asked what clothes are in your wardrobe, in your mind's eye you can take out each item and describe it. You can use this same skill to look at the tension spots in your body and to focus on reducing high blood pressure.

VISUALIZATION

The first step in using visualization is to take the time to examine mentally how your body feels. Do you have any pain or tension anywhere? Are you feeling stressed mentally? Next, imagine that you are able to visit the tension within your arteries and in some way get rid of it, perhaps by facing it down.

Take three slow, deep breaths right down into your abdomen and imagine yourself shrinking until you are small enough to travel through your arteries. Now, with your new, very small self, find a way into your own body, perhaps through the mouth, and set off on a journey of exploration. Think of your bloodstream carrying you toward any tense spots, gently and unhurriedly, but inexorably.

When you arrive, think about what the artery looks like. Is it blocked, or are the muscles constricted? Now look at the artery and consider what form or color it is. How do you feel about it? Are you resigned to it, angry and impatient with it, surprised to find it there at all?

Next, consider what would have to happen for the artery to get better. For example, you might consider dissolving the blockage bit by bit, scrubbing the artery walls, or thinning the blood. Finally, come back out of your body the way you went in and take a few deep breaths.

You may find this process a little strange and difficult initially. However, with practice you will be able to do it much more quickly and easily and be ready to start taking active steps toward relieving high blood pressure or using the technique to reduce tension anywhere in your body.

Find your place in the sun

A relaxation exercise called "Journey to the Golden Sun" can boost your circulation and sense of well-being. Lie down and relax completely by taking half a dozen slow,

FLOAT TO RELAX

Taking time out to float peacefully in a flotation tank can be an ideal way to let go of stress.

Little bigger than a bathtub, this totally enclosed, virtually soundproof tank is filled with water that is saturated with Epsom salts and kept at exactly skin temperature. The water feels neither warm nor cold and you can float effortlessly in it. No distracting light nor sound disturbs the imagination. Virtually all input to the brain comes via the sensory nerves. The flotation tank provides the ultimate relaxation experience, for some people, one that is perhaps even deeper than with meditation.

A session lasts one-half to two hours. The door can be opened from the inside if you wish to leave, but most people are surprised when it is opened at the end of a session. Some enthusiasts of the experience claim that when they come out of the tank, their senses are sharper and they have a heightened appreciation of the world around them. The effects of a single session may last for several days or weeks.

BACK TO THE WOMB
By mimicking the serenity of the womb, flotation tanks promote relaxation in a way that nothing else can approach.

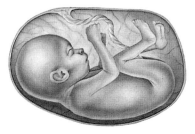

IDEAL STRESS RELIEF
Gradually allow your attention to drift to your body and how it feels. Become aware of each part of your body. Relax any areas of tension.

Wear a cap and ear plugs to protect hair and ears from salt.

deep breaths, right down to the bottom of your lungs. Each time you breathe out, hold for the count of three at the end and let all your tension drain away.

Then start to imagine a golden sun above you. In your mind, build up the picture until the sun is beautiful, bright, and warm. Imagine that a beam of light drops from the sun and picks you up. Your arms and legs are spread to let the sun fill your entire being with gold. Try to feel the energy going into your body. If you like, you can add a series of suggestions at this point. For instance, you might tell yourself: "I can feel the energy from the sun passing into my body, drawing all the energy it needs and soothing all my tensions. The sun's energy will revitalize my entire body, passing into every cell and every organ."

Stay in the light and warmth for as long as you like, and then return slowly with the sun's golden rays still coursing through your veins. Feel your blood overflowing with vigor and power.

Your own haven

A lot of people have their own "safe place" that they "visit" in their visualization exercises. You can find such a place for yourself. It could be a location you have actually been to or an entirely imaginary one: a beautiful beach, a hut in the mountains, or a clearing in a forest. Be creative when inventing your haven. Are there trees, a stream, a waterfall, a special seat to relax in or clothes that you like to wear while there?

Whenever you are feeling anxious or stressed about something, close your eyes and transport yourself to this place. If you are having problems with someone at work or with a personal relationship, take that person with you into the haven of your visualization exercise and imagine that you are sorting out the problem. This often has the effect of making you more relaxed around the person and creates a better atmosphere for resolving issues.

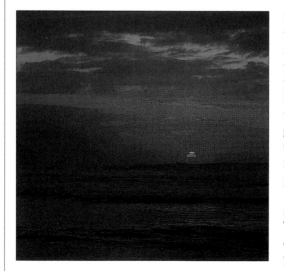

A QUICK ESCAPE
Visualizing an idyllic setting can be extremely relaxing and a good way to remove yourself from a stressful situation. Decide on your own ideal place and use it as your haven; move your mind there whenever you feel the need to relax.

POSITIVE THINKING

When you know how to relax your body, you are likely to find that negative moods disappear and that you have a sense of well-being and a more positive view of life.

To enhance your positive feelings about yourself and your life, take a moment to watch what is happening in your mind. Do you tend to get stuck in thought patterns that go nowhere? Do you feel helpless or powerless in some parts of your life? If you can sum up your negative feelings in one sentence, you can change your feelings into a positive statement that will support you and generate good feelings instead of bad. For instance, if you feel crestfallen when your boss finds fault with your work, you could try repeating to yourself "I am sensible and intelligent and good at my job." If you feel at a loss when dealing with a difficult family member, try saying: "I am patient, capable, and resourceful."

Just as repeated negative statements can undermine your self-esteem, so can positive thoughts generate good feelings. If you repeat these to yourself on a regular basis, you will soon begin to feel better about yourself. Write positive affirmations in large letters and stick them on your bedroom walls so that you see them as soon as you get up in the morning and just before you go to sleep at night. You may even want to make a tape of affirmations, repeating your positive characteristics over and over again.

Some people like to keep a journal to record both negative and positive thoughts. This is very useful for analyzing what kind of situations get you down and what makes you feel on top of things.

An extended stroll in the open air, a long, lazy soak in a warm bath, the absolute tranquillity of a flotation tank—these are ideal moments to explore and elaborate some positive statements about yourself and to begin your reprogramming for a more positive attitude about your life.

CHAPTER 5

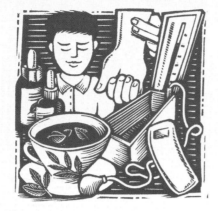

DIAGNOSIS AND TREATMENT OPTIONS

Symptoms of heart problems are an early warning to seek help. Techniques and equipment for investigating heart and circulatory disorders are better than ever and can usually provide an accurate diagnosis. Some natural methods provide further diagnostic tools that complement conventional ones, as well as offering treatment options to aid recovery.

SIGNS AND SYMPTOMS

Although some heart and circulatory diseases can do their damage silently, there are usually warning signs and symptoms that, if recognized early enough, could save your life.

First aid for an angina attack

Calmly help the person sit down and rest. If the patient has medication for angina, assist him or her in taking it. Should symptoms persist for more than 20 minutes after these measures, call for medical help.

A wide variety of symptoms accompanies both heart and circulatory diseases. Having one or more of these signs does not necessarily mean you have heart disease, but you should visit your doctor to rule out this or any other problem.

CHEST PAIN

Possible causes of chest pain that need to be ruled out before a diagnosis of heart disease is made include indigestion or heartburn (excess acid from the stomach), which can occur after eating; a strained muscle; a broken rib; a trapped nerve; inflammation of a rib joint; and lung infection (chest pain related to lung disease is usually most severe on breathing in). If, however, chest pain is due to coronary heart disease, the pain is

very distinct. It can be just a twinge or quite severe. The center of the chest feels very tight and heavy, or gripping, and this feeling may spread to the left or sometimes right shoulder, arm, neck, throat, or jaw. It usually lasts for 5 to 10 minutes, and angina medication sprayed into or sucked in the mouth can relieve it within a minute.

If attacks of chest pain last longer than 20 minutes or do not respond to medication, or if they recur over several days, seek medical help immediately.

Angina attacks

Angina pectoris, or simply angina, is the name given to pain that results from the narrowing of one or more coronary arteries due to atherosclerosis, which severely reduces the blood supply and oxygen delivery to the heart muscle. During exercise, stress, or emotional upset, the heart muscle has to work harder than usual and needs more oxygen to function properly, hence angina is usually brought on by these situations. Attacks are more likely when walking uphill or quickly, or when a person is tense or excited. In some cases, though, an attack of angina can come on while resting. Slowing or calming down usually eases the pain, and no permanent damage to the heart is done, although angina can signal that you are at risk of a heart attack.

Conventional treatment

A physician will carry out various tests, such as an exercise ECG (see page 93), to determine the severity of your angina and its causes, then he may prescribe drugs to prevent or treat the attacks. The doctor will also advise dietary changes, such as reducing fat intake, and management of stress. If your arteries are badly blocked, the doctor may recommend bypass surgery or balloon angioplasty (see page 111).

SYMPTOMS OF HEART DISEASE

The most common and immediate symptoms of heart disease are indicated here. Less common and more long-term symptoms include skin changes and changes in coordination and sensation.

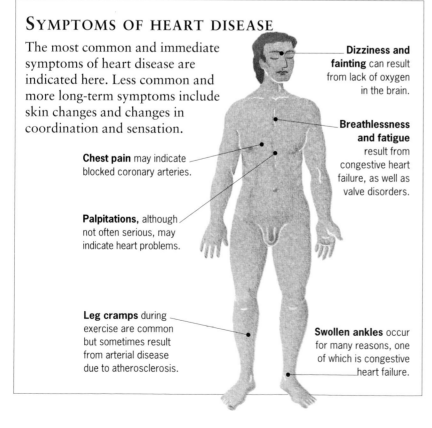

Dizziness and fainting can result from lack of oxygen in the brain.

Breathlessness and fatigue result from congestive heart failure, as well as valve disorders.

Chest pain may indicate blocked coronary arteries.

Palpitations, although not often serious, may indicate heart problems.

Leg cramps during exercise are common but sometimes result from arterial disease due to atherosclerosis.

Swollen ankles occur for many reasons, one of which is congestive heart failure.

Treating angina naturally

For regular sufferers of angina, a trained herbalist can help relieve symptoms. He or she may prescribe infusions (teas). Herbs said to help angina include hawthorn berry and lily-of-the-valley, which dilate the arteries, and motherwort, a relaxant that is believed to strengthen the heart. Other useful herbs include garlic, bromelain (from pineapple), and lime blossom, all of which have anticoagulant properties.

Acupuncture has long been used in China to treat angina, but orthodox doctors in the West do not recommend it as an exclusive treatment and suggest that it be used only in conjunction with prescribed medication. Acupuncture is beneficial for relaxation and pain relief, both of which make angina much easier to deal with.

Some natural therapists prescribe nutritional supplements, such as the antioxidant vitamins (see page 59), because these may help clear blocked arteries.

DIZZINESS AND FAINTING

Most attacks of dizziness—feeling lightheaded and unsteady for a few seconds—are not serious. Low blood pressure is a common cause. If these attacks recur frequently with no known cause, however, they could be an indication of heart or circulatory disease. Recurrent dizziness may be a sign that not enough blood is getting to the brain and that there may be blockage in an artery.

Fainting, also called syncope, is a temporary loss of consciousness due to a lack of oxygen reaching the brain. Again, fainting attacks are usually harmless and may occur simply because you have been standing for too long in a hot or stuffy atmosphere, such as a packed train. But in rare cases, fainting attacks could indicate a blockage in the heart, transient ischemia to the brain (temporary stroke) or heart rhythms that are too fast or too slow. Consult your doctor if you faint frequently.

PALPITATIONS

Fluttering or thumping sensations in the chest or neck are known as palpitations. You perceive your heart missing beats, beating rapidly, or thumping in the chest.

An emotional upset, stomach upset, exercise, fever, anxiety, and fear can all speed up the heartbeat and induce palpitations, and elderly people may experience palpitations

Pathway to health

Palpitations, even when harmless, can be unnerving, but certain herbs may help ease them. Particularly recommended are calming herbal teas, such as chamomile, valerian, bugleweed, and mistletoe (this last is also used to control blood pressure.)

Another herb often advised for palpitations is hawthorn berry, which is believed to help strengthen heart function. And night-blooming cereus is used for treating irregularities in heart rate and rhythm.

You should consult a trained herbalist or naturopath for treatment because herbs can be harmful when used improperly.

even without the above named stressors. Although palpitations can be very frightening, they are rarely serious and, unless they are persistent, should not cause concern.

Palpitations caused by heart disease, on the other hand, feel like the heart is beating very rapidly or very slowly, and they are usually accompanied by other symptoms, such as sweating, faintness, chest pain, and dizziness. These kinds of palpitations occur unexpectedly as a rule and are a sign that the heart's rhythm is seriously disturbed. A heartbeat that has an irregular rhythm or rate is called an arrhythmia and can have several causes.

Atrial fibrillation

This is an arrhythmia that occurs when the muscles in the atria do not contract together but instead flutter continuously, making the heart beat fast and irregularly. Atrial fibrillation causes palpitations and sometimes

WHAT TO DO IF YOU FEEL FAINT
Place your head between your knees and take deep breaths. If the feeling of faintness persists, lie down in a cool place, with plenty of fresh air, and elevate your legs on a cushion to restore blood supply to the brain. Loosen any restrictive clothing. Apply pressure to the acupressure point located two-thirds of the way between the middle of your top lip and your nose. Rest until you feel better. If breathing is difficult, get medical help.

Substances that cause palpitations
Many substances, such as certain prescribed drugs, nicotine from smoking, alcohol, and caffeine, can provoke a rapid heartbeat. This is rarely serious. However, if palpitations bother you, you may want to stop use of the responsible substance.

Ectopic heartbeats

Irregular, or ectopic, heartbeats feel like a missed beat or a thud in the chest because they originated in the wrong part of the heart instead of in the sinoatrial node, which normally regulates the heartbeat (see page 20). Though unnerving to most people, these heartbeats are not dangerous. Almost everyone experiences them once in a while, but they seldom require treatment. Excessive alcohol, caffeine, and tobacco are common causes.

chest pain, breathlessness, light-headedness, or fatigue. Blood in the atria does not flow normally, and clots may form. These can break free and cause a stroke, heart attack, or damage to other organs.

Tachycardia

When the heart beats too fast—over 100 beats per minute compared with a normal rate of 70 to 80—you may feel weak, become short of breath, and sweat a great deal. Most tachycardias are totally harmless. Occasionally, however, they are an indication that something is wrong with the ventricles (lower chambers of the heart), and serious injury to other vital organs, such as the brain, lungs, and liver, may result.

High or low concentrations of calcium, potassium, or magnesium (supplements of which are sometimes advised for people who have high blood pressure) can cause tachycardia. The levels of these minerals in the blood can also be affected by certain drugs, including diuretics. If you are taking any medication and experience palpitations, consult your doctor immediately.

Bradycardia

This is a very slow heartbeat. During sleep or at any time in super-fit people, the heart rate is usually slow. But when it goes below 50 beats per minute, a person may feel tired and dizzy; this could be a sign that something is wrong with the heart.

BREATHLESSNESS AND FATIGUE

During strenuous exercise it is quite normal to feel out of breath if you are unfit because the lungs can't keep up with the heart's demand for oxygen. But feeling breathless or extremely tired when you are at rest or doing low-intensity exercise may mean that your heart is not pumping properly or that its valves are faulty. In these cases, blood seeps back into the lungs, making them congested. Extreme fatigue may occur as tissues become starved for oxygen-rich blood.

Breathlessness and fatigue may simply indicate that you are stressed or run down or have a minor illness. If breathlessness occurs only at night, however, or when you are lying down, it may signal heart failure. To relieve breathlessness when lying down, prop yourself up on pillows. If breathlessness persists, consult your doctor.

LEG CRAMPS

When circulation of blood to the legs is partially or totally blocked due to a narrowing of arteries, the muscles do not get enough oxygen, and muscle spasms may occur. Leg cramps are quite common during strenuous exercise or when a person is unfit, but if you have them after a short walk or when you are walking very quickly or uphill and they stop as soon as you rest, you may have a leg arterial disease called intermittent claudication (see page 129).

Leg cramps caused by arterial disease may also be brought on by extreme cold or medication that causes the constriction of blood vessels. The location of the blockage in the arteries will determine which part of your leg becomes cramped. Consult your doctor if you have persistent cramps.

SWOLLEN ANKLES

Swelling, or edema, occurs when fluid leaks from the blood into tissues. Excess tissue fluid in the lower limbs can be the result of several conditions, including kidney damage, premenstrual fluid retention, starvation, and vitamin B deficiency.

EASING LEG CRAMPS

It is important to find out the cause of continued leg cramps because they may indicate arterial disease. To relieve the immediate discomfort, ask someone to massage your leg. If you have no one to assist you, take a warm bath to relax, then gently stretch your leg muscles and apply self massage.

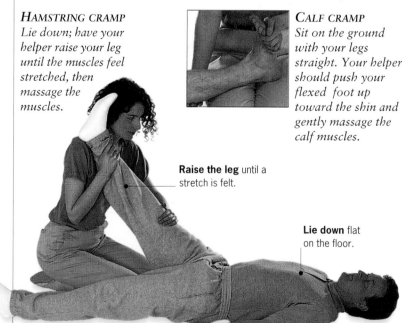

HAMSTRING CRAMP
Lie down; have your helper raise your leg until the muscles feel stretched, then massage the muscles.

CALF CRAMP
Sit on the ground with your legs straight. Your helper should push your flexed foot up toward the shin and gently massage the calf muscles.

Raise the leg until a stretch is felt.

Lie down flat on the floor.

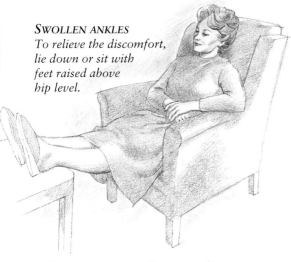

SWOLLEN ANKLES
To relieve the discomfort, lie down or sit with feet raised above hip level.

Gravity can contribute to edema, particularly in obese people. But even a person of normal weight can get swollen ankles from standing for long periods, hot weather, or a long journey on an airplane. A blood clot can cause edema if it blocks a vein. Some pregnant women and convalescents also suffer from swollen ankles.

Swelling may be attributed to heart failure when the heart is unable to pump blood out effectively and incoming blood backs up in the veins and leaks into tissues. Swelling in the ankles is the most common symptom, but fluid buildup can also cause abdominal discomfort and breathlessness. Consult a doctor if you have persistent swelling in the ankles and legs and if you have a family history of heart disease or other major risk factors. As a test, press the swelling. If a dent remains on the skin's surface (called "pitting edema") the swelling is more likely related to heart disease.

To relieve swollen ankles, wear loose, comfortable clothing. Support stockings may be necessary. Do not sit with your legs crossed and avoid standing still for long periods. To relieve swelling, sit or lie with legs raised above hip level. If you are traveling by airplane, walk up and down the aisle as often as possible. Cut down on salt because it can cause fluid retention. Gently massage your ankles to stimulate blood flow, using a massage oil such as tea tree or eucalyptus. Drink black tea or a diuretic herbal tea, like dandelion or corn silk.

SKIN CHANGES
Unusually white, bluish, reddish, or black skin or recurrent sores that do not heal may indicate cardiovascular problems. The usual cause is a blockage in arteries or veins.

SUDDEN CHANGES IN SENSES
Vision or speech disturbances, paralysis, weakness, and numbness may all indicate a stroke or transient ischemic attack (temporary stroke). These are usually the result of an arterial blockage from a clot that is impeding blood flow to the brain.

SHOCK
Shock is a combination of symptoms that include very low blood pressure, loss of consciousness (sometimes), cold and clammy skin, pale face, and poor breathing, all of which may be induced by a heart attack. If someone is in shock

▶ *Lay the patient down so the head is below the level of the heart.*

▶ *If the patient is not breathing, give mouth-to-mouth resuscitation (see page 116).*

▶ *Raise the patient's legs if this does not interfere with breathing.*

▶ *If the patient appears unconscious, place in a comfortable position on his or her side.*

▶ *Call for medical help immediately.*

HELP FOR A HEART ATTACK
The main warning sign of a heart attack is persistent, crushing pain in the center of the chest, which may spread to shoulders, neck, arms, throat, jaw, back, or abdomen. The person may also feel breathless, faint, sick, frightened, weak, or sweaty. An attack requires immediate medical attention and first aid if you can provide it.

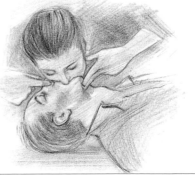

1 Call for medical help immediately if you suspect that someone is having a heart attack. Give the person an aspirin.

2 *Sit the person in a comfortable position if conscious and calmly reassure him. Loosen clothing.*

3 *If the person is unconscious and has stopped breathing due to cardiac arrest and you are properly trained, give cardiopulmonary resuscitation (see page 116). Otherwise, wait for medical help.*

DIAGNOSTIC TESTS

Some symptoms of heart disease are also those of less serious health problems. Doctors can use a range of tests to confirm or rule out a diagnosis of heart disease.

A doctor can learn a great deal about someone's heart just by doing a physical examination and paying careful attention to a description of symptoms. What is learned, together with the person's medical history and lifestyle risk factors, may indicate the presence of heart disease. But further tests are usually necessary for a precise diagnosis.

Listening to the heart through a stethoscope is a simple procedure, but it elicits valuable information if there are abnormal sounds that can indicate a heart disorder. All doctors are trained to do this. Special training, however, is required to carry out and interpret electrocardiograms, chest X-rays, Doppler echocardiography, radionuclide tests, CT and PET scanning, MRI, and cardiac catheterization (these are described on pages 94–95). Your symptoms will determine which tests you might need.

LISTENING TO THE HEART

The sound of the heartbeat is produced by the closing of the heart's four valves (see page 20). Using a stethoscope, a doctor will listen for abnormal sounds when the valves open and blood flows through them. If there is a a snap, click, or murmur, the valve may be damaged. For instance, a snapping noise indicates that a valve is abnormally narrow (stenosed). A clicking sound suggests that a heart valve is faulty; the click is caused by the sudden closing and opening of the abnormal valve. A murmur is a whooshing noise that is heard between normal heart sounds, when blood leaks back through a valve, passes through a narrowed valve, or enters the wrong part of the heart.

Doctors also listen for such other sounds as whoops, knocks, rubs, and gallops, all of which can indicate various abnormalities. As the murmur may change with position and breathing, your doctor will ask you to breathe in and out and adopt different positions in order to listen closely to your heart.

BLOOD TESTS

Analyzing blood and other body fluids provides further information about the heart. Blood tests are used to check the blood-cell count; oxygen, lipid, and enzyme levels; the presence of anemia (which may be made worse by heart disease); and clotting factors. Blood tests can also be used to assess the function of the kidneys and liver. Irregularities in these organs can be caused by damage as a result of heart disease.

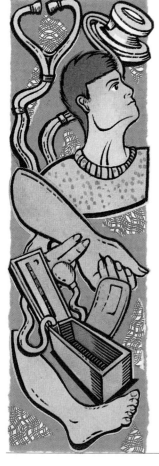

PHYSICAL EXAMINATION

During your physical examination a doctor or nurse will check the following:

SOUNDS

The doctor will listen to your breathing to hear if there is excess fluid in your lungs; to your heart for abnormal sounds; and to your blood vessels for whispering sounds that indicate obstruction.

VENOUS PULSE

The doctor will watch your jugular vein to see if the right heart chambers are pumping normally.

HEART RATE AND RHYTHM

The doctor will feel your pulse at various places to assess these. Places where the pulse is measured include the wrist, neck, groin, inner elbows, behind the knees, abdomen, and top of the feet and ankles.

BLOOD PRESSURE

Your blood pressure will be measured to get information on the pumping ability of your heart and arterial resistance. If your blood pressure is high, your heart will be overworking.

SWELLING

Your ankles, shins, thighs, lower back, abdomen, and hands will be checked for fluid retention.

HOMEOPATHIC DIAGNOSIS

Homeopathy uses dilute but powerful natural remedies to treat illness. It is a holistic therapy because it takes all aspects of the patient—body, mind, and spirit—into account. Because of this approach, homeopathy is very beneficial for overall well being, as well as for the health of the heart.

At the initial consultation a homeopath will ask you questions not only about your physical symptoms but also about your reactions to your job, other people, stress, the environment, and the weather; your moods, dreams, hopes, and fears; major events in your life; your childhood and adolescence; and any relevant family history. Based on all this information, a homeopath will arrive at a diagnosis and prescribe appropriate remedies.

It is always advisable to first seek the opinion of your doctor concerning the health of your heart, but homeopathy can complement the techniques of orthodox treatment.

Lipids

Your blood will be tested for low-density lipoprotein (LDL) and high-density lipoprotein (HDL) cholesterol levels as well as triglycerides (see page 53). Lipid tests are inaccurate by up to five percent so your doctor may test you on two different occasions. Most accurate results are achieved if you fast the night before a blood lipid test.

Enzymes

After a heart attack the damaged heart muscle releases cardiac enzymes into the bloodstream. Measuring the levels of these enzymes provides an indication of how much muscle has been damaged and also helps to narrow down possible diagnoses. It may take one to two days after a heart attack for these enzyme changes to be detected in the blood.

Oxygen levels

The oxygen content of your blood may be measured at different sites in your body, and blood may be taken from both veins and arteries. This will identify which part of the heart is not pumping blood adequately.

Clotting

Blood can be tested for the length of time it takes to clot. People whose blood clots abnormally quickly, and are therefore at risk of clots in their arteries, are sometimes put on medication to thin the blood.

ELECTROCARDIOGRAPHY

Electrocardiography (ECG) is probably the most frequently used test for diagnosing heart disease. Together with the exercise ECG (stress test), it is used for assessing all types of heart rate and rhythm disturbances and for distinguishing coronary heart disease from other types of heart disorders. It is a safe, quick, and painless test that records the electrical activity of the heart. Because no electricity goes into the patient from the machine, there is no danger whatsoever of getting an electric shock.

How an ECG works

Electrocardiography detects the flow of electricity through the heart that is associated with each heartbeat. The machine used in this test records the pattern of electrical impulses on a continuously moving strip of paper or a monitor. The image it produces is called an electrocardiogram. Different waves on the graph represent electrical impulses as they travel to different parts of your heart.

If the heart muscle has been damaged, the electrical impulses then become altered and an abnormal pattern is detected.

During the test, the person either sits or lies down. Electrodes (gel pads) are taped to each of the arms and legs and to six places on the front and left side of the chest. Jelly is placed on the skin where the electrodes are attached to ensure good contact. These electrodes are connected by 12 wires to the ECG machine, which amplifies the electrical impulses before recording them.

What the ECG is used for

A standard ECG test is generally used to pick up abnormalities of heart rhythm and to identify defects in the conduction of electrical impulses through the heart. It can also detect old and recent heart attacks and indicate whether the heart is enlarged or not pumping properly.

The standard ECG test, however, does have its limitations. Sometimes it shows abnormalities when the heart is healthy. At other times it suggests nothing is wrong

ECG readings
Electrocardiograms provide useful information about the heart. Three of the readings below show different heart problems.

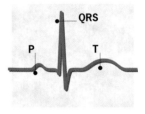

This ECG graph shows a normal heartbeat with regular P, QRS, and T wave patterns (see box, page 21).

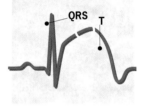

The peak between the QRS complex and the T wave indicates that a heart attack is occurring.

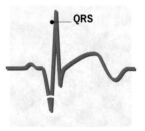

The deep part of the QRS complex shows that a heart attack might have occurred in the past.

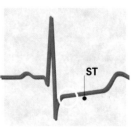

The lowered ST segment suggests that the heart is not receiving enough blood, and angina may be occurring.

An Airline Pilot at risk

A middle-aged man's risk of heart disease is greatly increased if his lifestyle includes some unhealthy habits and if there is a history of heart disease in his family. He should have any symptoms that signify heart problems checked out immediately and take action to minimize all risk factors.

Alan, a 38-year-old commercial airline pilot, is married to Judy, who looks after their two young children, Caroline and David. His compulsory annual checkups have not yet revealed any physical damage from his steady diet of airline food and excessive drinking on occasion to help him unwind from the stress of flying, but the company doctor has advised him to stop smoking.

For the past month he has felt at various times an uncomfortable pain in his chest, which lasts a few minutes. Alan is concerned because he is slightly overweight and does not exercise regularly. His father and grandfather had heart attacks in their fifties, and he and Judy fear he is suffering from angina. They are really worried he will lose his job.

WHAT SHOULD ALAN DO?

Alan must see his doctor and find out the cause of his chest pain as soon as possible. If there is any suspicion of heart disease, he has to inform his company and cannot continue to work as a pilot until a firm diagnosis is made.

He and Judy should discuss the possibility that he may have to change jobs and be prepared for dealing with this situation.

Alan must realize that he needs to lead a healthier life, regardless of the current condition of his heart. He has to quit smoking, improve his diet, lose weight, exercise regularly, and reduce his stress levels by learning relaxation techniques. Alan should also reduce his alcohol consumption substantially.

Action Plan

FAMILY
Talk to Judy about plans for the future in terms of job and family. Perhaps Judy could work part-time for a while.

WORK
Inform company about undergoing medical tests. Arrange for vacation leave to relax and recover from the examinations.

HEALTH
Stop smoking and drink less. Eat more fruits and vegetables and less fat. (Take along fruit and other healthful snacks for long trips.) Join a yoga class to relieve stress.

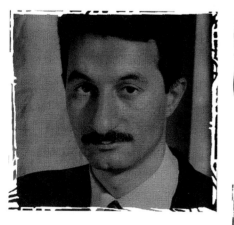

WORK
When loss of a job is threatened by heart disease, stress is compounded and may worsen symptoms.

FAMILY
A family history of heart disease greatly increases a person's risk for it and is a source of concern.

HEALTH
Stress, smoking, high alcohol consumption, poor diet, and lack of exercise are all preventable risk factors for heart disease.

HOW THINGS TURNED OUT FOR ALAN

Alan's general practitioner sent him for an electrocardiogram (ECG) and exercise ECG, neither of which showed any heart abnormalities. However, in view of his family history, the doctor referred Alan for a coronary angiogram. The test was normal, ruling out heart disease. The GP concluded that Alan's chest pains were due to stress. On her suggestion, Alan took a vacation and started doing relaxation exercises. He also quit smoking and cut down on his drinking.

with the heart when there actually is. Further testing will confirm the results. False readings occur at random, although they can also be affected by medications that the patient is taking. The ECG is therefore most useful to confirm suspected heart disease, but it is always interpreted in context, that is, in the presence of heart-related symptoms.

Exercise ECG (stress test)

A standard ECG test is not wholly efficient at diagnosing conditions related to insufficient blood supply, like angina, which are most likely to occur during exercise or periods of unusual or prolonged stress. The exercise ECG, also known as stress testing, was developed to improve diagnoses.

The patient is monitored with electrodes (as in the regular ECG), while walking on a treadmill or pedaling a stationary bicycle. The exercise begins at a leisurely pace but becomes harder and harder. Blood pressure measurements are taken at various times during the test.

The test ends when the patient experiences pain, becomes really tired or very short of breath, or significant changes are recorded by the ECG. On average, the test takes 15 to 30 minutes.

Although exercise testing is an improvement on a standard ECG, it is not 100 percent accurate and is more inaccurate for women than men for unexplained reasons.

Holter (ambulatory) ECG monitoring

This is a continuous ECG recording that is used to detect intermittent abnormal heart activity. It is useful for diagnosing palpitations. The person being tested wears a portable device called a Holter monitor for 24 hours, while going about his or her everyday activities (except taking a bath or a shower). Recording leads are stuck to the front of the chest and wires are connected to the attached monitor. The person being tested has to keep a diary to record times and types of activities. Changes on the ECG can then be interpreted in the light of when certain activities occurred.

IMAGING TECHNIQUES

There are many different ways to observe, or look at, the heart—its shape and size, pumping action, the flow of blood in and out of its chambers, and the size and shape of its valves. These techniques will show up structural abnormalities and help a doctor make a correct diagnosis.

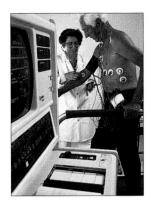

*EXERCISE ECG
Because angina is often
exercise-induced,
exercise ECGs are
commonly used to test
for it. The test is quick
and noninvasive.*

TRADITIONAL CHINESE MEDICINE

Traditional Chinese medicine takes a holistic view of health, looking at the body as a system in which all the parts work in harmony. The main focus is prevention rather than cure, but a wide range of treatments is available when things go wrong. These include acupuncture, dietary changes, herbs, massage, and exercise programs. The practitioner of Chinese medicine has four main methods of making a diagnosis:

▶ *Looking at the person's general appearance, complexion, and tongue and listening to the voice. The tongue is examined for unusual colors and bumps. (On different areas of the tongue these may indicate problems with certain organs of the body.)*

▶ *Taking notes on and considering the patient's medical history, including family history and lifestyle factors.*

▶ *Smelling for unusual body odor, breath, and excretions.*

▶ *Feeling the pulse at both wrists, the abdomen, at meridians (invisible lines that store chi, or energy, and connect the body's organs) and at the acupuncture points.*

The practitioner uses a pulse diagnosis to assess the health of various body organs and the flow of *chi*, or the life force, that passes through and around them. When there are blockages in the path of the life force, the body becomes more prone to illness. Acupuncture releases these energy blockages and restores the flow. The pulse assessment is the Chinese doctor's most important tool in the diagnosis of heart problems.

Through acupuncture, Chinese medicine can successfully treat both high blood pressure and angina, as well as help to relieve stress. It is believed that acupuncture stimulates the production of the body's own pain-killing hormones, called endorphins.

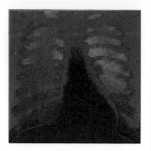

HEALTHY HEART
This colored X-ray shows a heart with a normal shape and size (the red pear shape in the center).

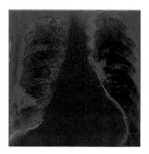

ENLARGED HEART
The heart in this X-ray (the large pear shape bulging to the right of the picture) is abnormally enlarged due to hypertension. This condition could lead to heart failure and other complications.

ECHOCARDIOGRAPHY
Ultrasound is used to create an image of the heart through a computer. It can show the shape and size of the heart muscle, as well as valve disorders and congenital heart disease.

CHEST X-RAY

This is usually the first imaging technique a doctor uses. It is quick and painless and shows the size, shape, and position of the heart. A chest X-ray can detect if the heart is enlarged and confirm that it is failing to pump properly. The picture can also reveal calcium deposits in the coronary arteries, valves, and heart muscle, and can see the condition of the lungs (fluid in the lungs indicates possible heart failure).

ECHOCARDIOGRAPHY

This is a safe and painless test that is based on ultrasound. High-frequency sounds are transmitted onto your internal organs by the scanning head, called a transducer. They are then reflected back into the transducer, which converts the echo into electrical signals. The pattern created by the sounds is interpreted by a computer and displayed on a screen. Using this technique, it is possible to get an image of the moving heart. Echocardiography is used to investigate disorders of heart valves, congenital heart defects, and heart muscle shape, size, and blood-flow patterns.

During the test, the person lies on his or her back or side. Gel or oil is rubbed onto the chest to improve sound-wave transmission, and the transducer is moved around the chest. The echoes picked up form a picture on a nearby monitor screen.

Specialized echocardiography

A special technique, Doppler echocardiography measures the speed of the blood flow in different parts of the heart. One of its principal uses is for transesophageal echo-

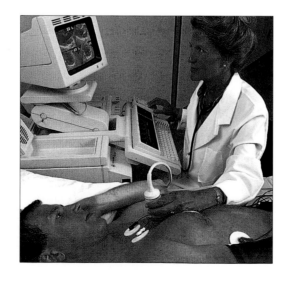

cardiography, which makes it possible for pictures of the heart to be taken from the esophagus (the tube that runs from the throat to the stomach). Because the esophagus lies directly behind the heart, a more detailed view can be seen from it.

The ultrasound transducer is attached to a tube, which is then passed down the esophagus. A short-acting sedative is given to the patient in order to relax the muscles and minimize discomfort.

RADIONUCLIDE TESTS

These tests are more specialized than the ones discussed so far. A small and harmless amount of a radioactive substance (an isotope), such as thallium or technetium, is injected into the bloodstream, where it is carried through the circulatory system to the heart. There, it is detected by a gamma camera, which picks up any emitted radioactive rays. The isotope decays rapidly, so the dose of radioactivity someone receives is very small—about the same as that received when undergoing a chest X-ray.

During radionuclide tests, pictures are generated through a computer and show the heart's chambers as they empty and fill with blood. Images of the blood flow to the heart muscle can also be obtained. This test may be done while the person is stationary or while exercising on a treadmill, as with the exercise ECG.

Types of scanning

Two types of radionuclide scanning are used to look at the heart: thallium scanning and technetium scanning. Thallium is used to study the blood flow to the heart muscle. Technetium is used to test the size and pumping activities of the heart chambers to assess how well the heart is ejecting blood, thus establishing the efficiency of the heartbeat.

The risk of damage to the patient from the tiny amount of radioactive material used is extremely slight. But nuclear scanning is not used, as a rule, with women who are pregnant or breastfeeding.

Radionuclide scanning is time consuming, expensive, and requires more special equipment and specially trained staff compared with ECG and echocardiography. It may sometimes be necessary, however, to obtain more detailed information than is supplied by other tests of the blood and oxygen supply to the heart.

POSITRON EMISSION TOMOGRAPHY (PET) SCANNING

PET scanning, which gives much better resolution than radionuclide scanning, is particularly useful for predicting whether someone will recover after a heart attack or benefit from a coronary artery bypass. It is also used to check impaired blood flow.

The patient is first given a mild sedative, then a radioactively tagged substance (usually carbon, nitrogen, or oxygen) is injected into a vein. From there the gas travels to the heart and is taken up by the muscle cells. Positively charged particles, or positrons, that are emitted by the radioactive gas cause the release of tiny quantities of gamma rays. An image created from these rays by a computer show the activity that is going on in different parts of the heart muscle, thus revealing how the muscle is using energy.

RAPID COMPUTED TOMOGRAPHY (CT) SCANNING

This produces pictures of the heart muscle when X-rays are passed through the body at different angles. A computer-generated image provides a much more detailed picture of the heart than a conventional X-ray because it can show where the heart muscle is failing during the pumping cycle.

The patient lies on a table that slides inside a large X-ray machine. The machine directs X-rays in cross sections through the person's body. Occasionally a contrast material may be injected into a vein to make the image clearer. There is very little risk in this procedure.

MAGNETIC RESONANCE IMAGING (MRI)

This technique provides a high-quality image of the heart and major blood vessels without the use of radiation. It is very useful for diagnosing congenital heart defects. The patient lies on a table that slides inside a large magnetic machine (a newer version is open on the sides), where radio waves are passed through the chest. The machine detects energy signals given off by atoms of body tissues, which are constructed into an image. MRI pictures are similar to X-rays but show more detail.

There are no risks associated with MRI, but people who have pacemakers or other internal metallic objects that may cause interference cannot undergo the procedure.

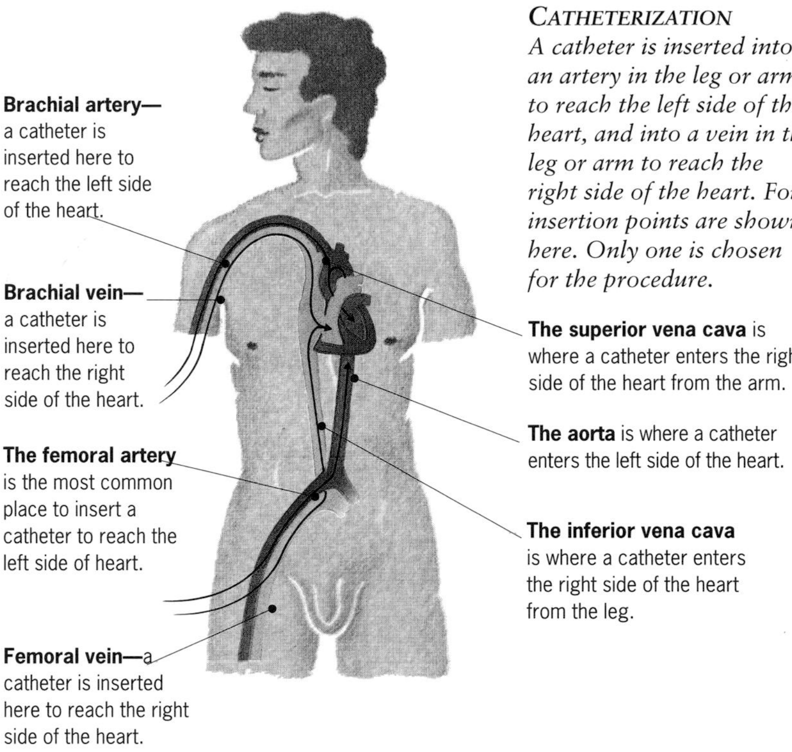

Brachial artery— a catheter is inserted here to reach the left side of the heart.

Brachial vein— a catheter is inserted here to reach the right side of the heart.

The femoral artery is the most common place to insert a catheter to reach the left side of heart.

Femoral vein— a catheter is inserted here to reach the right side of the heart.

CATHETERIZATION
A catheter is inserted into an artery in the leg or arm to reach the left side of the heart, and into a vein in the leg or arm to reach the right side of the heart. Four insertion points are shown here. Only one is chosen for the procedure.

The superior vena cava is where a catheter enters the right side of the heart from the arm.

The aorta is where a catheter enters the left side of the heart.

The inferior vena cava is where a catheter enters the right side of the heart from the leg.

CARDIAC CATHETERIZATION

This procedure is used to investigate the heart's pumping ability, valve efficiency, and any coronary artery blockages. A long flexible tube, called a catheter, is used. It may be fitted with a minute measuring device, or dyes may be injected through it into the heart.

Under a local anesthetic, a catheter is inserted into the groin or the arm and is threaded through a vein or artery up into the heart. X-ray screening is used to make sure the catheter is placed in the heart correctly.

After the catheter is properly inserted, an electrocardiograph monitors the heart continuously for about 45 minutes. You do not actually feel the catheter in the heart. When the test is over, the catheter is removed. Occasionally, a few stitches are needed where it was first inserted. The test is performed with an empty stomach, and some medication may be given beforehand. The whole procedure takes about an hour.

Variations

The catheter may have a special device on the end to measure oxygen levels in the blood, blood pressure in arteries or heart chambers (balloon flotation catheters), or electrical impulses in different areas of the heart (electrode catheters).

continued on page 98

Balloon flotation catheter
This special kind of catheter is often used to measure blood flow and pressures in the ventricles of the heart and pulmonary artery. A catheter with a small balloon on the tip is inserted into a vein or an artery. When it reaches the heart, the air-filled balloon enables the catheter to move through the heart, propelled by the blood flow, while a device inside it monitors blood pressure. The catheter is often left for a few days in order to monitor heart function continuously.

Home Tests

You can assess your health with do-it-yourself cholesterol and blood pressure measuring kits, a heart rate monitor to measure your response to exercise, and simple tests for checking whether or not your weight is within healthy limits.

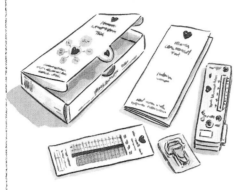

CHOLESTEROL SELF-TESTING KITS
These kits can be useful for people who are trying to lower their cholesterol level and want to check on it periodically without making a trip to the doctor's office. However, the kits measure only total cholesterol, and a laboratory test should still be done periodically to assess levels of HDLs and LDLs (see page 52).

Blood pressure and cholesterol self-testing kits can be bought in many pharmacies and health food stores. For most adults, a blood pressure reading under 140/90 indicates there is nothing to worry about, and purchasing a kit may be an unnecessary expense. It is enough to have blood pressure checked once a year by a doctor. But a self-testing kit for use at home may be useful for someone who has been diagnosed with borderline high or high blood pressure and wishes to monitor it more often.

With some home blood-pressure monitors, all you have to do is place a finger on a sensor, which displays a blood-pressure reading.

Other more complex, but less expensive, types involve wrapping a cuff around your arm and automatically or manually inflating it and reading the pressure on a gauge.

Bear in mind that blood pressure can fluctuate with stress, emotional upset, and illness, so if a reading is high, make a note of it and measure again in a few days.

CHOLESTEROL KITS

Many self-testing kits can give a cholesterol reading in minutes from a finger-prick sample of blood. When performing a cholesterol test, be sure to read and follow the instructions carefully and bear in mind that blood cholesterol levels vary from day to day. They can also be affected by general state of health, the time of day, whether or not you have been fasting, even the time of year (possibly being higher in winter).

If you have had a minor illness, such as a cold or the flu, you should delay testing for about three weeks. If you have suffered a major illness, delay the test for about three months or until you are fully recovered. If your level is high, you may want to do a second test to confirm this result and possibly even a third test.

Kits usually register total cholesterol levels. A blood cholesterol level below 200 mg/dl (milligrams per deciliter) is desirable; 200–239 mg/dl

is borderline high risk; 240 mg/dl and over is considered high. If your test results are high, you can help lower them by following a diet low in saturated fat and high in soluble fiber and eating lots of vegetables and

fruits, which are usually high in the antioxidant vitamins (A, C, and E). Exercise is also an important factor. If such measures do not yield a lower reading, drug therapy may be necessary. Talk to your doctor.

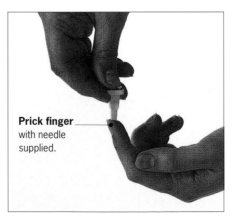

Prick finger with needle supplied.

1 *Prick your finger with the needle provided. Bear in mind, if you squeeze your finger too hard, more plasma—the clear part of blood—will come out and you will get an inaccurate reading.*

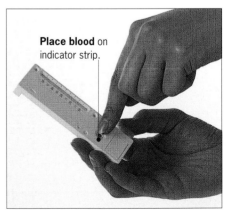

Place blood on indicator strip.

2 *Place your finger on the indicator strip provided and put blood on the spot indicated in the instructions. Wait for a few minutes (as specified) and then compare your reading with the key.*

MEASURING YOUR PULSE

During aerobic exercise it is important to monitor heart rate (heartbeats per minute). You can get a fairly accurate measurement by taking your pulse To measure it, halt or slow down your movement and find the pulse at the neck or wrist (see below and right for the locations). Watching the second hand on a watch, count the heartbeats for 10 seconds, then multiply this number by 6 to determine your rate per minute. Halfway through your regimen the rate should be within your target zone (see page 70).

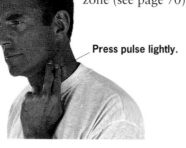

Press pulse lightly.

NECK PULSE (CAROTID ARTERY)
"Draw" a line from the base of your ear to the top of your breast bone. At about the midpoint along the line, just under the jaw, press two fingers against your neck until you feel a pulse. (Do not press so hard that you block the flow of blood, or you will not feel a pulse.)

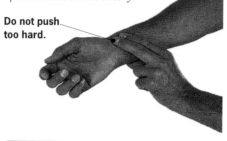

WRIST PULSE (RADIAL ARTERY)
Place two fingers (index and middle) between the bone and tendon that lie just under the ball of the thumb and press gently until you feel the pulsing of the blood in the artery.

Do not push too hard.

ARE YOU OVERWEIGHT?

The chart below gives the ranges of normal weights for men and women at different heights. Check to see if you are in the normal weight range. Your age and build determine which end of the range you should be in—the lower end is for younger people. If you are concerned about being either underweight or overweight, consult your doctor or a nutritionist for advice on changing your diet. Also, see page 62 for a healthy heart diet.

You may wish to embark also on a more regular exercise program because this will help burn up additional calories. See page 142 for the approximate number of calories you need per day to maintain your present weight. To lose pounds you must eat fewer calories than you burn.

HEART-RATE MONITORS

If you have a diagnosed heart problem, you may want to use a heart-rate monitor when doing aerobic exercise; it will tell you if you are exceeding your target heart rate zone (see page 70)—a potentially dangerous situation.

The heart-rate monitor shown below consists of electrodes mounted on an electronic transmitter and attached to the chest with an elastic belt. It picks up electrical impulses from the heart and sends them to a wrist monitor, which looks like a watch. Both the chest band and the wrist monitor are lightweight and comfortable.

IDEAL WEIGHT CHART

Check your weight against your height. The figures for women's heights include 5-cm (2-in) heels; men's include 2.5-cm (1-in) heels.

HEIGHT	MEN (acceptable weight)	WOMEN (acceptable weight)
1.57 m (5 ft 2 in)		46–59 kg (102–131 lb)
1.60 m (5 ft 3 in)		48–61 kg (105–134 lb)
1.63 m (5 ft 4 in)	54–67 kg (118–148 lb)	49–63 kg (108–138 lb)
1.65 m (5 ft 5 in)	55–69 kg (121–152 lb)	50–64 kg (111–142 lb)
1.68 m (5 ft 6 in)	56–71 kg (124–156 lb)	52–66 kg (114–146 lb)
1.70 m (5 ft 7 in)	58–73 kg (128–161 lb)	54–68 kg (118–150 lb)
1.73 m (5 ft 8 in)	60–75 kg (132–166 lb)	55–70 kg (122–154 lb)
1.75 m (5 ft 9 in)	62–77 kg (136–170 lb)	57–72 kg (126–158 lb)
1.78 m (5 ft 10 in)	64–79 kg (140–174 lb)	59–74 kg (130–163 lb)
1.80 m (5 ft 11 in)	65–81 kg (144–179 lb)	61–76 kg (134–168 lb)
1.83 m (6 ft)	67–83 kg (148–184 lb)	63–78 kg (138–173 lb)
1.85 m (6 ft 1 in)	69–86 kg (152–189 lb)	
1.88 m (6 ft 2 in)	71–88 kg (156–194 lb)	

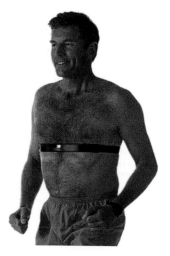

HEART-RATE MONITOR
Read instructions carefully before using your monitor.

SEEKING A SECOND OPINION

After you have been diagnosed by your doctor, you may wish to seek a second opinion if

▶ *The diagnosis is very serious.*

▶ *The proposed treatment is extensive, risky, or experimental.*

▶ *Surgery is suggested.*

▶ *There is a choice of treatments and you are unsure which one is best for you.*

▶ *You do not feel happy with the information your doctor has supplied.*

▶ *You do not have confidence in your doctor for any reason.*

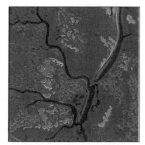

*CORONARY ANGIOGRAM
This test is used to assess arterial disease resulting from atherosclerosis, and is used also to see blood clots. Dye is injected via a catheter and an X-ray of the heart is taken. Here, a blockage is seen in one of the coronary arteries, where the red dye is broken.*

Catheters are also used for treatment procedures, such as angioplasty, which helps to clear blocked arteries (see page 111), and valvuloplasty, which opens narrowed valves (see page 117).

Serious complications of catheterization are very rare, but there may be bruising in the groin or a weakened pulse in the arm.

ANGIOGRAPHY AND VENOGRAPHY

Certain procedures can be used along with catheterization to make the investigation of blood vessels clearer and to reveal blockages and clots in vessels. In angiography, a dye is injected through a catheter into an artery. X-ray pictures are then taken of the dye's flow through the artery. Venography is based on the same principle, only the dye is injected into a vein to show any blockage.

In coronary angiography, opaque dyes are injected into the chambers of the heart or coronary arteries via a catheter. These structures can then be seen more clearly on a monitor. This is the most common way to examine the extent of atherosclerosis.

In left ventriculography, a dye is injected into the left ventricle of the heart to show its pumping efficiency or any leakage.

With these procedures a small number of people experience nausea or vomiting after injection of the dye or, even more rarely, an allergic reaction to the dye itself.

MAKING A DECISION

Diagnostic tests can be exhausting and stressful, and the outcome may be rather frightening, presenting you with a decision to make about treatment and changes in your habits. It is important to realize, however, that no diagnostic test is 100 percent accurate, no matter how carefully it is done. One test cannot be expected to give the whole answer, but each one should supply information that will lead the doctor to the correct diagnosis, when all the factors are taken into consideration.

If you have been diagnosed with a heart problem, you need to make sure you understand exactly what the disorder is, how it was caused, and what the prescribed treatment is, in order to make the correct decision to improve your health.

If you want a second opinion, ask your primary care practitioner for another referral and inform the first specialist that you have decided to go for a second opinion.

A NATURAL APPROACH

You may have decided with your doctor about the medical options for treatment, yet you still feel that something is missing. There are natural therapists who take a different approach to the diagnosis and treatment of illness. They typically pay attention to the whole person—including body, mind, emotions, and spirit—unlike conventional doctors, who may concentrate mainly on the physical symptoms. A naturopath, homeopath, practitioner of traditional Chinese medicine, an aromatherapist, or an herbalist may give you some insight into causes of your illness and suggest methods you can use in addition to your medical treatment to aid your return to health.

An alternative therapist will ask detailed questions about every aspect of your life. These will be similar to questions asked by your doctor, including your symptoms; information on previous illnesses, accidents and hospitalizations; chronic illnesses and allergies; illnesses that run in the family; results of any previous medical diagnostic tests; and lifestyle habits, such as smoking.

Depending on the diagnosis and which therapist you have consulted, you will be given various treatments. The naturopath, for instance, will typically advise dietary changes, exercise, herbal remedies, and relaxation techniques. A homeopath will prescribe very dilute but potent extracts from natural remedies. An aromatherapist may suggest the use of massage and various oils for relaxation and stress relief. A traditional Chinese doctor may use acupuncture (see page 101) to relax you, lower your blood pressure, and relieve pain, and herbal remedies to dilate the arteries and stimulate the heart's contractions and the circulatory system in general. There are many herbs with medicinal properties that a trained herbalist can administer with great effect to relieve your symptoms.

No matter what the diagnosis or what treatment course you take with your doctor or surgeon, it is important to see your body as inseparable from your lifestyle and make any necessary changes in your habits to improve your health.

Conventional and alternative medicine can be combined to achieve the maximum benefit, as long as the doctors and therapists involved are informed of all the treatments you are undergoing.

NATURAL TREATMENT OPTIONS

You can accelerate your recovery from heart disease with natural therapies, which range from acupuncture and herbal medicine to yoga and meditation.

Many doctors who practice conventional medicine also recommend natural remedies to their patients who have heart and circulatory diseases. Voicing feelings, avoiding stress, sleeping well, exercising more, and eating healthily not only are natural but also form a major part of every heart disease recovery plan.

HYDROTHERAPY

Any therapeutic approach based on the use of water is called hydrotherapy. It can improve circulation, ease joint and muscular pain, and aid relaxation. It is often prescribed by naturopaths.

Warm baths
To calm the body generally and lower blood pressure, a warm bath with lavender oil added to it is recommended.

Cold showers
To stimulate heart and circulatory function, take a cold shower for just a few seconds daily. This treatment, however, should not be undertaken by elderly or sick people.

Circulation in the legs can be improved by pouring cold water on them, particularly below the knees, every morning.

Swimming
Swimming regularly provides an excellent cardiovascular workout and can help prevent some heart disorders. It is also a therapeutic exercise for recovering heart and stroke patients. Caution: Hydrotherapy should always be practiced under the supervision of a trained therapist.

Natural therapies, also called alternative or complementary therapies, embrace many approaches that can be useful in fighting heart disease. Practices like yoga and meditation ease the mind and help relieve stress; others, such as acupuncture, act directly on body tissues; still others, such as the Feldenkrais Method (see page 144), can help you relate more closely to your body's needs.

Some natural approaches, used by people around the world for centuries, are simple and can be done at home, while others require the aid of a trained therapist. Most doctors do not object to treatments that offer physical or psychological benefits with few, if any, risks or side effects attached.

FINDING A BALANCE

Before using a natural therapy, discuss your plans with your doctor. Certain herbal medicines, for instance, might cause a bad reaction when taken with a medication your doctor is prescribing. You should also talk to your doctor before taking up a movement-based therapy, such as yoga or t'ai chi, so he can advise you of any restrictions that might be necessary. Similarly, you should give a natural therapist complete details of your medical history, symptoms, and habits. These will influence the choice of treatment.

With the cooperation of your doctor, it may be possible to combine conventional and natural medicines that complement each other. For example, if you are told to give up smoking, you might want to use acupuncture to help you stop. Herbal teas might help you get the sleep you need without taking drugs. Relaxation exercises and meditation can also be useful in getting to sleep or in reducing your stress level. More unusual approaches, like laughter therapy

The success of natural therapies
Some people believe that an important reason for the effectiveness of these therapies is the amount of attention paid to the patient by the practitioner. Being allowed to talk about your concerns with a sympathetic listener is, after all, good therapy, and it will almost certainly make you feel better.

THE KNEE JET
Spraying cold water on the legs to improve circulation has been a popular hydrotherapy treatment since the 1800s.

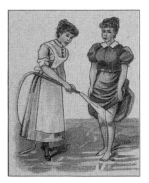

HOW TO FIND A THERAPIST

Below are some ways you may find a therapist. Once you have done so, check the therapist's professional qualifications. Ask how long the person has been practicing. Above all, heed your instincts. A natural therapist should be someone you like, trust, and can confide in.

► *Contact the professional organization that represents the therapy and request a list of local practitioners.*

► *Ask a practitioner of another therapy for a recommendation. People in health-related fields often know one another.*

► *Ask your doctor.*

► *Check the yellow pages for listings of therapists or of natural health centers.*

► *Get recommendations from friends.*

► *Check notices at your local health food store.*

or crystal healing have made some people feel better and certainly do no harm, as long as conventional treatment is sought as well.

In fact, most natural therapies pose no danger to health, as long as you use them with your doctor's knowledge and approval. It is, however, particularly important not to stop taking any medication without first discussing the possible consequences with your physician.

HEALING THE BODY

Many natural therapies aim to treat specific physical symptoms and generally improve physical health. Several of these also have the added benefit of healing the mind.

Naturopathy

In the 19th century some physicians recommended a cure in which the body was stimulated to heal itself. Known as the Nature Cure, its only prescriptions were healthy (whole) food, exercise, clean air, and water. Naturopaths still follow this tradition today, although most are not as restrictive in their

approach and believe that the body often needs additional help to heal itself. Naturopathy (see page 122) is multidisciplinary, focusing mainly on diet, nutritional supplements, exercise, hydrotherapy (see page 99), relaxation exercises, and herbal remedies. Some naturopaths also practice homeopthy, acupuncture, and/or massage. Naturopaths refer patients to orthodox practitioners when there is a clear need for surgery or drugs.

Aromatherapy

In this therapy essential oils extracted from plants are used to treat specific disorders. It is based on the idea that individual aromas or mixtures of them have therapeutic effects; also that certain oils can be beneficial when absorbed through the skin. For instance, lavender is often used to calm anxiety and relieve stress. Aromatherapy can aid relaxation and thereby help lower blood pressure. Massage that makes use of essential oils can improve the circulation. An aromatherapist is qualified to advise you on the most appropriate oil for your needs.

MASSAGE FOR HEALTH

Massaging the body, particularly with aromatherapy oils, is very conducive to relaxation and can help reduce high blood pressure. Back and face massages are particularly good for relieving stress.

Massage can also bring relief from leg cramps (see page 88), which may occur as a result of arterial disease. Fluid retention, which can result from congestive

heart failure, and also certain valve diseases may be relieved by a vigorous body massage. However, you should check with your doctor before having a vigorous massage to be sure you are well enough for it. Massage provides good stimulation for anyone's circulatory system and can help to prevent such disorders as varicose veins.

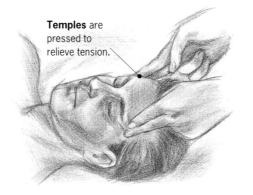

Temples are pressed to relieve tension.

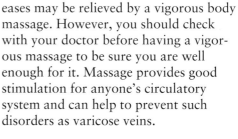
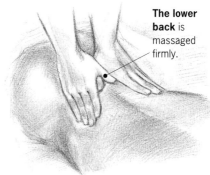

The lower back is massaged firmly.

FACE MASSAGE
A massage therapist may use long, stroking movements on the face or press on various pressure points, particularly around the eyes, where many people hold tension.

BACK MASSAGE
To start, long, firm strokes will be used to warm the muscles, then firmer pressure will be applied on tense spots, followed by cupping and chopping to stimulate the circulation.

Oils can be used in different ways, but most are potent and must be utilized in very small amounts. To use in a bath, add a teaspoon to the running water. To make an inhalation, add a few drops of your chosen oil to a basin of boiling water, place a towel over your head, then hold your face over the basin and breathe deeply for 2 minutes. For an aromatherapy massage oil, add 2 drops of essential oil per teaspoon of base massage oil. Base massage oils include almond, wheat germ, and sunflower, which are available in health food stores.

Acupuncture and acupressure

Based on an ancient Chinese system of stimulating certain energy points in the body, both acupuncture and acupressure can aid in recovery from illness and restore the body's natural energy balance. For acupuncture, needles are used to stimulate these points, while for acupressure, finger or hand pressure is firmly applied.

According to theories of Chinese medicine, acupuncture works by regulating the

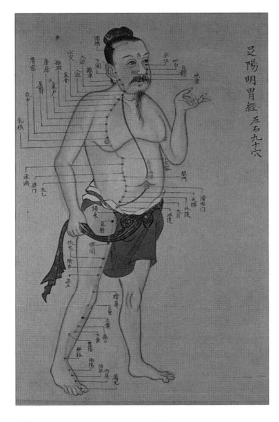

ACUPUNCTURE MERIDIANS
This ancient Chinese diagram shows some of the critical points for treatment with acupuncture. These points lie on meridians, lines along which chi—the life force—flows.

life force known as *chi*. Too little chi causes weakness, while blockages preventing its flow through the body can cause illness. Chi is believed to flow along 12 invisible lines known as meridians; these connect the body's internal organs where the chi is stored. An acupuncturist increases or unblocks the flow of chi by inserting very fine stainless steel needles along the meridians at particular points, thereby relieving symptoms. There are more than 1,000 of these points in the body, each of which is thought to have a different effect.

In the treatment of heart disease, both acupuncture and acupressure can be used to stimulate circulation and provide relief from high blood pressure and angina. While conventional doctors may not agree about treating heart problems with these methods, they generally accept that both acupuncture and acupressure are often successful in relieving pain, inducing relaxation, reducing stress, and overcoming addiction. However, doctors explain these effects as resulting from the stimulation of points that release endorphins, which are the body's natural pain-killing hormones.

Acupuncture can be carried out only by a qualified therapist, but you can perform acupressure as a self-help remedy. It is best to ask a practitioner to advise you on the pressure points relevant to your illness (a few points are illustrated in Chapter 6). To be of lasting benefit, acupressure needs to be done at least three times a week for about an hour each time. You should be in a relaxed, comfortable position before you start. Use your finger and press firmly but not too hard. This pressure should be maintained on the relevant point for several minutes at a time.

If you are using these techniques on someone else, always be gentle with older people or anyone who is ill or very upset. Avoid doing acupressure on anyone who is intoxicated or has just eaten.

Herbal medicine

Every culture in the world has used plants to treat illness, and the effectiveness of herbal remedies is being given ever more attention today. Like synthetic drugs, however, herbs can be dangerous if they are used incorrectly. One of the most widely used and well-known heart drugs, digitalis, which has been used for over 200 years to treat heart failure, comes from the leaves of

Moxibustion
Some acupuncturists use moxibustion in combination with needles or instead of them to treat high blood pressure. For this procedure the downy coverings of the leaves of the herb *Artemesia moxa* are gently burned above an acupuncture needle. Alternatively, the moxa may be rolled into a stick and held, lighted end down, just above the skin over the relevant acupuncture point.

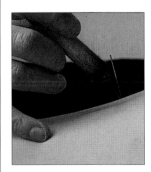

MOXA STICKS
Made from the herb, Artemesia moxa, burning moxa sticks may be used to relax tense back muscles, relieve stress or pain, and help lower blood pressure.

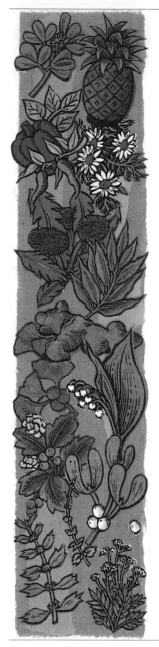

HERBS AND YOUR HEART

A wide range of herbs can benefit the heart and circulatory system. You can drink them as teas, apply them as lotions or compresses, or simply use them in cooking. Caution: medicinal quantities of herbs are powerful and should be taken only under the supervision of a qualified herbal practitioner.

HERB	FUNCTION
Alfalfa (*Medicago sativa*)	Acts as a mild diuretic; may help lower cholesterol.
Balm, or lemon balm (*Melissa officinalis*)	Promotes relaxation; may calm palpitations brought on by anxiety.
Bishop's Weed (*Ammi Visnaga*)	Relieves angina and palpitations; improves coronary circulation.
Bromelain (pineapple) (*Ananas comosus*)	May relieve symptoms of angina; breaks down blood clots.
Buckwheat (*Fagopyrum esculentum*)	Used in folk medicine to relieve edema and prevent arteriosclerosis.
Bugleweed (*Ajuga reptans*)	May make the heart beat more slowly.
Chamomile (*Chamaemelum nobile*)	Promotes relaxation; helps relieve stress and anxiety.
Cayenne (*Capsicum frutescens*)	May help dissolve blood clots and lower cholesterol.
Dandelion (*Taraxacum officinale*)	Acts as a mild diuretic.
Garlic (*Allium sativum*)	Lowers cholesterol; prevents clots; may prevent arteriosclerosis.
Ginger (*Zingiber officinalis*)	Helps lower cholesterol; makes platelets less sticky; stimulates blood circulation.
Ginkgo (*Ginkgo biloba*)	Improves circulation; helps prevent blood clots.
Hawthorn (*Crataegus oxycantha*)	Improves coronary circulation; reduces high blood pressure by dilating arteries and reducing cholesterol buildup; strengthens heart muscle; normalizes arrhythmia.
Lily-of-the-valley (*Convallaria majalis*)	Improves general heart function and normalizes arrhythmia.
Mistletoe (*Viscum album*)	Reduces high blood pressure; helps prevent buildup of plaques in arteries; strengthens capillary walls; helps relieve anxiety.
Motherwort (*Leonurus cardiaca*)	Strengthens the heart; normalizes arrhythmia; helps relieve anxiety. (Pregnant and nursing women should avoid it.)
Night-blooming cereus (*Selenicereus glandiforus*)	Dilates blood vessels; normalizes arrhythmia.
Onion	Helps reduce cholesterol; acts as an anticoagulant.
Skullcap (*Scutellaria lateriflora*)	May help lower blood pressure; relieves stress and anxiety.
St. John's wort (*Hyperium perforatum*)	Relieves stress and anxiety; aids relaxation.
Valerian (*Valerian officinalis*)	Relieves stress and anxiety; aids relaxation.

the foxglove plant. The leaves themselves, however, are poisonous; just because a substance is natural does not mean it is safe. You can buy many dried herbs and herbal preparations in health food stores, but if you have a serious illness it is always best to consult a qualified medical herbalist, preferably with the knowledge and support of your own doctor.

Herbalism can offer a wide variety of benefits to an ailing heart. Proponents claim that certain herbs, taken in the right dosages and combinations, act as natural diuretics, lower cholesterol, improve circulation, and even dissolve blood clots. Some plants used in herbal remedies, including garlic, ginger, and onion, are foods as well as herbs and therefore pose no health risks. Many studies have shown that all three are instrumental in lowering cholesterol levels and other blood fats, as well as reducing high blood pressure.

Some herbal preparations are taken as teas; others, in such forms as poultices and ointments, are applied to the skin. Herbalists often recommend heart tea (see opposite) for slowing down a fast heartbeat. People who react intensely to stressful situations and get palpitations may find it calms them and soothes their nerves, but anyone who has been diagnosed with arrhythmia (see page 114) should consult their doctor before taking it. Hawthorn berry tea, drunk daily, is also recommended as a preventative against heart problems. Although herbs can be a useful addition to a healthful lifestyle, it should be noted that lifelong damaging habits cannot be overcome by using them.

Homeopathy

By treating sick people with tiny doses of substances that would cause the same symptoms of the disease in a healthy person, homeopaths claim to cure many illnesses. This theory and the principle behind it of treating "like with like" has been advocated since the time of the ancient Greeks. It was turned into the formal system of medicine known as homeopathy by a German doctor named Samuel Christian Hahnemann (1755–1843). Paradoxically, the more diluted the medication is, the stronger its action. Hahnemann wrote: "The power to heal is released so that even a totally inert substance can come to influence the vital force."

Some scientists assert that the doses in homeopathic remedies are so small that they are worthless in a therapeutic sense, yet about half of the practitioners in the United States are physicians who recognize their effectiveness. Most doctors have no objection to their patients taking homeopathic remedies, as long as they themselves are informed of their use and their patients continue with conventional medical treatment.

Although homeopathic remedies can be bought in many health food stores and pharmacies, treatment of any serious condition, such as heart disease, should be undertaken with a qualified homeopath because the remedies do not have the same effects on everyone. However, some over-the-counter remedies may bring relief of symptoms.

HEALING THE MIND

A large part of recovering from a heart attack or major surgery takes place in the mind. Studies have shown that a positive mental outlook is a good aid to recovery.

Heart tea
Mix two parts mistletoe, two parts motherwort, four parts balm leaves, four parts St. John's wort, and eight parts hawthorn leaves and blossoms in a teapot. Pour boiling water over the herbs, leave to steep for 5 to 10 minutes, and then drink two to three cups as needed.

HERBAL PREPARATIONS

Your herbalist will advise you on which herbal preparation best meets your needs.

Infusions, or teas, are made with the leaves, flowers, and/or stems of herbs, depending on where the active ingredients are found. To prepare a tea, pour 450 ml (2 cups) boiling water over 70 g (2½ oz) of chopped fresh herbs or 30 g (1 oz) of

chopped dried herbs and cover. Let stand for 10 to 15 minutes and then strain.

Decoctions are made with the roots or bark. To prepare, add 60 g (2 oz) of chopped fresh herb or 30 g (1 oz) of crushed dried herb to 750 ml (3 cups) cold water, bring to a boil, and simmer until liquid reduces to 500 ml (2 cups). Cool, then strain through a plastic sieve.

To make a poultice, crush or pound fresh or dried herbs and mix with enough hot water to form a paste. Spread liberally on a strip of cloth, preferably cotton, and apply to the skin.

HAWTHORN BERRY INFUSION
This infusion may improve your circulation and help clear out arteries. Drink a cup three times a day. To sweeten the infusion, add a little honey.

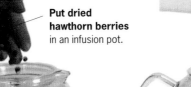

Put dried hawthorn berries in an infusion pot.

Pour boiling water over the berries.

Steep infusion for at least 10 minutes before drinking.

BREATHING MEDITATION

This is a very relaxing and soothing meditation, often taught to beginners. Sit in a comfortable position in a quiet place, with soft light (candles create a pleasant atmosphere).

▶ *One: count each inhalation until you reach 10. Start again, and keep repeating for about 3 minutes.*

▶ *Two: count each exhalation until you reach 10; repeat for about 3 minutes.*

▶ *Three: focus on each whole breath, consciously noting its movement into your lungs, then out again. Do this for about 3 minutes.*

▶ *Four: concentrate on the point at which breath first enters your body—at the edge of your nostrils. As you inhale, feel life and energy entering with it. Repeat for about 3 minutes.*

▶ *Five: sit quietly to absorb the relaxing effect of this meditation.*

Therapies that work on the mind can also help the body recover by aiding relaxation and reducing tension.

Meditation

One of the oldest techniques for achieving control over the mind is meditation. This takes a variety of forms, which include silent contemplation on a word, phrase (mantra), or image; chanting; and counting breaths. To obtain the best results, try to meditate for 10 to 15 minutes both morning and evening. (See page 36 for "humming meditation" and the box, right, for "breathing meditation.") Meditation may also include visualization (see page 83). Many people who suffer from high blood pressure have found that meditating has greatly reduced, even eliminated, their need for prescription drugs.

Yoga

A series of slow stretches and breathing exercises that deeply relax the mind and body, yoga is an excellent way to reduce tension and manage stress The practice also improves flexibility, mobility, circulation, and muscle strength. It can also effectively relieve pain, but learning which posture to do for a specific source of pain requires the help of a qualified instructor.

Yoga has been proven very effective in lowering high blood pressure and because it also reduces stress, it is a particularly good choice of exercise for someone with heart disease. Also, it can be performed by people of any age or fitness level.

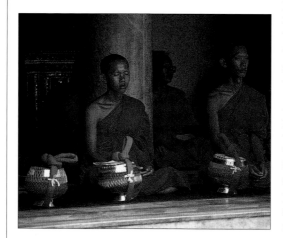

MEDITATION
Religious groups around the world have long used meditation as part of a way of life. Buddhists (shown above) believe that you should meditate at least once a day for a healthy mind.

YOGIC BREATHING FOR HIGH BLOOD PRESSURE

Lie down on the floor and place one hand on your abdomen and the other on your chest. Inhale slowly, at the same time pushing out your abdomen, then slowly exhale, feeling your abdomen deflate. Pay attention to the hand on your chest; there should be very little movement there. Repeat the procedure for several minutes. This exercise teaches you to breathe deeply, which is essential for stress management. It relies on minimal effort for a maximum intake of oxygen.

In the mid-1980s, Dr. Dean Ornish, an American cardiologist and director of the Preventive Medicine Research Institute in Sausalito, California, started using yoga for relaxation and blood pressure reduction as a component of his program for treating heart patients. His patients were also advised to follow a low-fat vegetarian diet and to walk for 30 minutes every day. Some 82 percent of the people in this program showed some degree of reversal of arterial disease in their follow-up angiograms. The patients who made the most progress in reversing heart disease were the ones doing the most yoga—1¼ hours twice a day.

Biofeedback

Very effective in helping to control blood pressure, biofeedback (see page 141) allows individuals to gain control over such functions as brain waves and blood pressure by teaching them the power of concentration and relaxation with the help of machines that are sensitive to body functions.

Hypnotherapy

Both physical and psychological complaints can be treated with hypnotherapy. A hypnotist aims to induce a state of deep relaxation in the patient in order to make positive suggestions: for example, to give up smoking or let go of stress. If the patient is receptive, hypnosis can be very effective for changing habits, learning to cope with stress, giving up addictions, and relieving pain. It is also possible to learn to hypnotize yourself. Autogenic training (see page 42) is a popular form of self-hypnosis.

CHAPTER 6

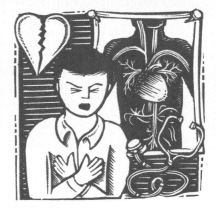

HEART AND CIRCULATORY DISORDERS

*The heart and circulation can be
afflicted with many different disorders
that have a wide variety of causes; these are
sometimes unavoidable but most often are linked to
lifestyle. Conventional medicine is almost always the
primary method of diagnosis and treatment, but
natural therapies can play a part in relieving
symptoms and aiding in recovery.*

HEART DISORDERS

A healthy lifestyle can go a long way toward warding off many types of heart disorders. However, some problems, like congenital heart disease and certain infections, may be unavoidable.

Congenital heart disorders

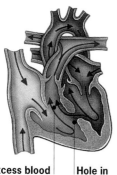

Excess blood to lungs | **Hole in septum**

HOLE IN THE HEART
A hole in the septum between the ventricles results in too much blood flowing to the lungs.

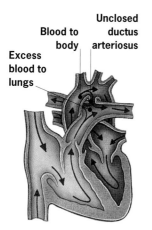

Blood to body | **Unclosed ductus arteriosus**

Excess blood to lungs

PATENT DUCTUS ARTERIOSUS
Oxygenated blood is pumped from the aorta back to the lungs instead of to the rest of the body.

There are a number of different heart disorders, each with its own set of causes, symptoms, and treatments. In some cases natural therapies can be used in conjunction with conventional treatment and may help to ease symptoms or aid in recovery. Because many heart disorders can be serious or life-threatening, it is wise to check with your doctor before embarking on a course of natural therapy to be sure it will not conflict with your medication.

CONGENITAL HEART DISORDERS
About one percent of babies are born with a congenital heart disorder—that is, one that is present from birth. The heart is one of the first organs to develop, starting as a single, pulsating tube with arteries at one end and veins at the other. Between the sixth and twelfth week of gestation, often before the mother even realizes she is pregnant, this tiny tube folds back on itself to develop the basic structures of the mature heart. During these crucial weeks the heart is particularly vulnerable to damage.

If a mother contracts a viral infection like rubella (German measles) in these early weeks, there is an increased chance that her baby's heart will develop abnormally. Alcoholism in pregnant women can cause a heart murmur in the fetus. Most congenital heart disorders, however, have no known cause and are not hereditary, although some defects are slightly more common in twins. Some disorders are minor enough not to require treatment; others are life threatening.

There are many types of congenital heart defects, but they can all be divided into two main categories: those that cause too much blood to flow through the lungs and not enough around the body, and those that result in too little blood reaching the lungs, and therefore too little oxygen in blood flowing around the body.

Hole in the heart
A common problem is a structural abnormality known as hole in the heart. The name refers to a hole in the septum (partition) between the chambers of the heart, and it may occur between the ventricles (ventricular septal defect) or the atria (atrial septal defect). These two defects account for 50 percent of all congenital heart problems. Both result in too much blood flowing to the lungs, which leads to breathlessness and exhaustion from any kind of exertion. A small hole does not require treatment; a large hole is corrected with surgery, usually between ages 5 and 10.

Patent ductus arteriosus
The second most common congenital heart condition, patent ductus arteriosus accounts for 5 to 10 percent of such problems. It occurs when the passage (ductus arteriosus) between the pulmonary artery (to the lungs) and the aorta does not close after birth. This results in excess blood flowing to the lungs, causing breathlessness and possibly infection of the heart lining. Sometimes the defect can be corrected with drug treatment. Otherwise, surgery is performed before the child is five.

Transposition of arteries
The two most important blood vessels of the heart, the pulmonary artery and aorta, may be transposed, with the pulmonary artery growing from the left ventricle instead

DID YOU KNOW?
Folic acid is essential for development of the nervous system, but excessive quantities can cause an abnormally slow fetal heart rate. Although pregnant women are often advised to a take folic acid supplement, they should not ingest megadoses of it.

FALLOT'S TETRALOGY

A complex disorder that results from a combination of four different abnormalities, fallot's tetralogy occurs in one out of every 2,000 births and accounts for 10 percent of all congenital heart disorders. The valve in the pulmonary artery is narrowed; there is a hole in the wall between the two pumping chambers of the heart (a ventricular septal defect); the aorta is abnormally large and in the wrong place; and the muscular wall of the right ventricle is abnormally thick and inflexible. The result is that much of the blood circulates to the body without being oxygenated in the lungs, causing a "blue baby." Corrective surgery is vital and is usually done as soon as the child is strong enough to withstand open-heart surgery, usually before the age of five. A child who has had successful surgery can usually lead a normal life.

of the right and the aorta from the right instead of the left ventricle, so oxygenated blood goes to the lungs and deoxygenated blood to the body. This results in a "blue baby," whose skin, lips, and nails have a bluish pallor. Immediate surgery is needed; another operation is usually necessary during the child's first 18 months.

Heart valve disorders

Various problems can occur with the valves, one-way doors at the entrance to the pulmonary artery and the aorta respectively that control the flow of blood in and out of the heart chambers (see pages 115–118). These disorders can be caused by a congenital birth defect, as well as an infection or disease of the heart later in life.

Narrowing of a heart valve is a common problem. A narrow opening forces the heart to pump too hard as it tries to push blood through. The limited blood flow caused by a narrowed valve can result in a variety of problems, including congestive heart failure and heart rhythm disorders. A valve that does not close properly is another concern. It will allow some blood to flow back in the wrong direction, setting the stage for infection, abnormal heart rhythms, and clotting.

Treatment of either condition may not be necessary, but the heart should be moni-

tored regularly. For more severe problems, drug treatment may be prescribed or a damaged valve repaired or replaced.

Diagnosis

Some abnormalities can be detected before birth when the mother is given an ultrasound scan. This safe and painless technique is performed using high-frequency sound waves to build up a picture of the baby's development in the uterus.

If serious abnormalities are detected, then a staff of medical specialists can be on hand at the birth to provide immediate, and often life-saving, care (see page 108). But some disorders become apparent only after birth, when a baby may turn blue, have labored breathing, or collapse suddenly.

Sometimes congenital heart disorders become apparent only toward the end of the child's first year of life or even remain undetected until preschool or school medical checkups, when strange heart sounds or an unusual pulse rate alert the doctor.

Several different procedures, either singly or in combination, can then confirm the diagnosis. These include X-ray examination and an electrocardiogram, or ECG (see page 91), cardiac catheterization (see page 95), and echocardiography (see page 94).

Treatment

If a defect is minor, then an operation might not be necessary, but severe abnormalities can be corrected only by surgery. Fortunately, many congenital disorders actually heal themselves in time. Half of all holes in the heart close up by themselves during infancy and only about one-third of children born with heart defects need surgery.

FATIGUE
A child with a heart problem is often tired and irritable and needs a lot of rest.

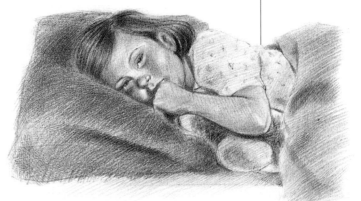

Breast-feeding and heart defects
Years ago breast-feeding was discouraged for babies with congenital heart disorders because it was believed that doing so would tire them out too much. We now realize, however, that babies actually use less energy and breathe more efficiently during breast-feeding than during bottle-feeding. Also, breast milk can protect the baby from infections because it contains the mother's antibodies. Small, frequent feedings are recommended.

LIFESTYLE AND ATHEROSCLEROSIS

As with any heart or circulatory disorder, there are a number of lifestyle changes that are essential to prevent further damage from atherosclerosis. These include:

▶ *Losing weight, if necessary, and reducing cholesterol levels with a low-fat diet that includes lots of fresh vegetables and fruits.*

▶ *Quitting smoking (see page 36), and minimizing intake of alcohol and caffeine.*

▶ *Exercising regularly.*

▶ *Practicing relaxation and stress management techniques (see page 150).*

▶ *Lowering blood pressure (see page 43).*

ATHEROMA
This image showing a cross-section of an artery reveals a thick deposit of fat, which causes atherosclerosis.

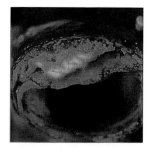

TREATMENT IN THE UTERUS

Doctors are now attempting to treat some life-threatening congenital heart disorders before a baby is born. A procedure called balloon angioplasty is being used in some cases to widen narrowed aortic valves and is meeting with a fair amount of success. The aortic valve is the one-way valve situated at the exit of the left ventricle in the aorta. If it does not open properly, the ventricle is unable to pump enough oxygenated blood around the body.

The procedure involves inserting a catheter into the heart of the fetus through the abdomen and uterus of the mother, using ultrasound for guidance. The catheter, which is only one millimeter wide, has a tiny balloon at one end that is carefully positioned in the narrowed aortic valve and gently inflated, pushing the valve open.

When surgery is needed, doctors prefer to correct the whole problem at one time to minimize disruption to the child's life. But it is sometimes necessary for a child to have two operations, an early one to remedy the worst of the defect and prevent further damage from occurring, and another when he or she is older, and hopefully stronger, to complete the repair. In very few cases, when defects cannot be totally corrected, treatment will consist of minimizing symptoms and helping the patient live as long and comfortable a life as possible.

Outlook

The prognosis varies, depending on the type of disorder, the age when it is discovered, the degree of damage, and the success of the treatment. Many children go on to lead normal and healthy lives. However, even after surgery, problems can still surface, including an irregular heart rhythm and endocarditis, infection of the valves or endocardium (see page 117), both of which require regular medical observation.

Extra care must be taken to avoid all infections. The child will have to be given antibiotics before any dental or medical procedure and be kept away from children who have infections. Also, the child needs a healthy diet and plenty of rest.

Natural therapies

There are no natural therapies that can be recommended for congenital heart disease, because the defect needs to be corrected.

ATHEROSCLEROSIS

Atherosclerosis, or hardening of the arteries, is caused by the buildup of fatty deposits. These first appear as fatty streaks, often where arteries branch off. As the streaks become bigger, the artery walls become damaged and calcium deposits, called atheromas or plaques, form. Platelets, red blood cells, blood fats, and fibrin (a protein involved in clotting) accumulate on plaques, making them bigger. This reduces the diameter of arteries and makes artery walls less flexible, further increasing blood pressure. With the high blood pressure itself or physical exertion, plaques may crack and cause the artery wall to bleed. A blood clot then forms that reduces blood flow further, causing angina or intermittent claudication (see page 129); or blood flow may become totally obstructed, causing a stroke or heart attack.

Atherosclerosis usually occurs in middle-aged and elderly people, as arteries thicken and stiffen with age. It is most common in men in their forties, but after menopause women are just as susceptible. Factors contributing to atherosclerosis include smoking, high blood pressure and cholesterol levels, a sedentary lifestyle, family history of heart disease, diabetes, and obesity. Stress is also a major factor because the stress hormones cortisol and adrenaline increase production of triglycerides (a fat in body tissue) and cholesterol, as well as the stickiness of platelets.

Symptoms and diagnosis

The symptoms and diagnosis will depend on the cause and location of the diseased arteries. Atherosclerosis causes angina if it occurs in the coronary arteries (see page 110), stroke if it occurs in the brain arteries (see page 127), and intermittent claudication if it occurs in the leg arteries (see page 129).

Treatment

The most important step is to quit smoking. It is also essential to reduce blood cholesterol by following a low-fat, high-fiber diet and increasing intake of fresh vegetables and fruits. Blood pressure must also be lowered (see page 23). Medication to reduce cholesterol or blood pressure may be prescribed.

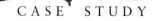
A Child with a Hole in the Heart

The causes of congenital heart disease are not usually known, although infection in the mother or environmental factors may play a part. Surgery is sometimes necessary, but most children with congenital heart disease recover and lead healthy lives. It is very unusual for a family to have more than one affected child.

Karen and Mark were delighted when Louise was born. She seemed healthy at birth, but in her checkup at six weeks old, a doctor found that Louise had a heart murmur. She was then given a chest X-ray, electrocardiogram, and echocardiogram. (Louise had to be sedated for the echocardiogram to stop her wriggling.) She was diagnosed as having an atrial septal defect (a hole in the bottom part of the septum) and a leaky mitral valve. No treatment was required for the mitral valve, but Karen and Mark were told their daughter would need an operation at age five to repair the hole. Louise is now five and is small for her age. She is not able to play with her friends for long periods because she tires easily.

WHAT SHOULD MARK AND KAREN DO?

Mark and Karen need to prepare Louise and themselves for the operation. They should talk to Louise about going to the hospital, try to explain what will happen with pictures and games, and if possible, take her to visit the hospital beforehand. They can be encouraging by telling her she will be able to play with her friends when she gets better.

Karen and Mark should make sure they understand the whole procedure and how to deal with it. They also need to overcome their understandable but unjustified feelings of guilt that they were in some way responsible for Louise's defect, in order to give her the love and support she needs to fully recover.

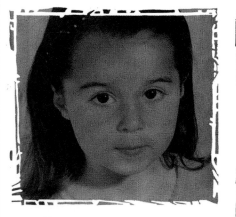

EMOTIONS
Having your newborn baby diagnosed with heart disease is traumatic and often causes feelings of grief, anger, and guilt.

HEALTH
A child with a congenital heart defect may suffer breathlessness, fatigue, and poor weight gain.

LIFESTYLE
A baby with a heart defect has a good chance of survival, but special care is needed to prevent infection.

Action Plan

EMOTIONS
Join a support group at the hospital to discuss grief and fear. Get as much information as possible.

HEALTH
Watch Louise closely for fatigue or breathlessness. Make sure she does not get overtired or catch a cold, and that she has a healthy, balanced diet.

LIFESTYLE
Take care to prevent infection, and if one develops, consult the doctor immediately so that antibiotic treatments can be started. Tell Louise's dentist, school, and friends' parents about her condition.

HOW THINGS TURNED OUT FOR LOUISE

Karen and Mark joined a parent support group run by a cardiac center. Louise was admitted to the hospital and had a 4-hour operation. She was allowed to go home after 10 days. For the first few weeks she was tired and irritable, but soon regained her energy. After six months Louise started taking part in normal activities. In the future she will have to take antibiotics before any medical procedures to prevent the chance of infection.

HEART AND CIRCULATORY DISORDERS

DISEASED CORONARY ARTERIES

Several physical conditions can affect the health of coronary arteries and result in angina, heart muscle damage, or even a heart attack. Stress, too, can lead to coronary spasm, which may temporarily cut off blood flow to the heart.

EXTENT OF DAMAGE
Irreversible damage to the arteries results only from complete obstruction of the blood supply.

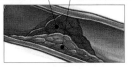

Blood clot   **Atherosclerosis**

Blood clot and atherosclerosis in a coronary artery may cause a heart attack.

Damage to muscle is caused by blood clot blocking blood supply.

Atherosclerosis

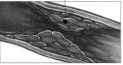

Spasm

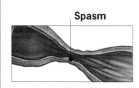

Spasm in a coronary artery restricts blood supply to muscle.

Blood supply to muscle is only partially restricted by spasm or atherosclerosis.

Atherosclerosis in coronary artery restricts blood supply to the muscle.

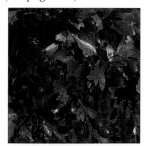

HAWTHORN
The flowers, leaves and berries of this shrub (Craegus spp.) have been used by herbalists for over a hundred years to treat heart disorders. A hawthorn berry infusion is recommended for clearing out arteries and improving circulation (see page 103).

If the atherosclerosis is well advanced, balloon angioplasty (see page 111) may be performed. This surgical procedure pushes the plaque apart and widens the artery, but the measure often needs to be repeated within a couple of years. Laser catheters may also be used (see page 111).

Natural therapies

Certain natural therapies can help limit the damage caused by atherosclerosis, and some may actually reverse it. Naturopaths recommend taking supplements of the antioxidant vitamins A, C, and E (see page 59) to prevent oxidation of "bad" (LDL) cholesterol, which causes fatty deposits in arteries. Important catalysts for the actions of these vitamins include zinc (found in liver, fish, and eggs), manganese (in nuts, cereals, and egg yolks), selenium (in vegetables and seafood) and vitamin B_6 (in cereals and meat).

Some fats actually help prevent atherosclerosis, including the omega-3 oils found in fish. Other sources of omega-3 include flaxseeds and flaxseed oil, evening primrose oil, black currant seeds, and borage.

Herbalists recommend eating bromelain (contained in pineapple), which breaks down fibrin (protein in clots), and garlic, onion, and ginger, which help reduce blood cholesterol as well as thin the blood to reduce the risk of clots. Soybean products and peanut oil may also help reduce cholesterol.

Some herbs are helpful when taken as teas or capsules. These include hawthorn berry, to dilate the arteries, and mistletoe, to help prevent the buildup of plaques.

Because stress hormones increase production of cholesterol, reducing stress is essential for lowering cholesterol levels. Aromatherapy oils, such as lavender and lily of the valley, can be used as part of massage or in baths to enhance relaxation. Relaxation or visualization exercises (see page 83), meditation (see pages 36, 104), and autogenic training (see page 42) are all helpful.

ANGINA AND CORONARY HEART DISEASE

When the coronary arteries are damaged due to atherosclerosis, blood clots, or spasm of the artery walls, the blood supply to the heart is restricted and angina results. Angina (see page 86) is chest pain that occurs as a symptom of coronary heart disease, also called coronary artery disease. If the coronary arteries become totally obstructed, then a heart attack (myocardial infarction) may occur (see page 112).

Angina occurs whenever the heart's workload exceeds the ability of the coronary arteries to supply it with blood. This blood starvation of muscle is called ischemia. Angina nearly always disappears with rest because the demands on the heart are lessened, and the coronary arteries can again meet the heart's demand for blood. The pattern of angina tends to be predictable, although trigger factors vary from one individual to another. However, if the pattern changes for the worse and attacks become more frequent and/or more severe for over three months, a heart attack will occur in one-third of cases unless action is taken.

Medical advice from a specialist should always be sought if angina is suspected, and if a diagnosis is made, individuals will have to make changes in habits, diet, and causes of stress. Natural remedies can also be helpful to relieve some of the symptoms.

Diagnosis

Doctors use several procedures to diagnose angina and coronary heart disease, including standard and stress ECG (see page 91), echocardiography (see page 94) and nuclear scanning techniques (see page 94).

If such tests indicate that there are problems with the supply of blood to the heart, a more sensitive procedure is needed to discover exactly what is going on and where troublesome narrowing of the arteries has occurred. A doctor may then advise coronary angiography (see page 98).

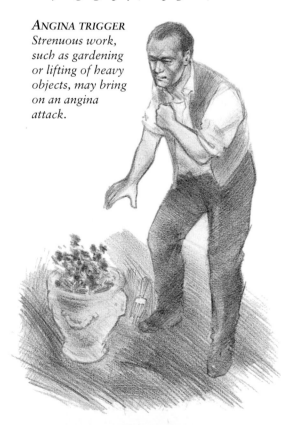

ANGINA TRIGGER Strenuous work, such as gardening or lifting of heavy objects, may bring on an angina attack.

Treatment

If the coronary arteries are not seriously impaired, then treatment will aim to help the sufferer adopt a healthier lifestyle to lower blood pressure and heart rate. In more severe cases, however, drugs may be used to reduce the heart muscle's workload. Drugs are also prescribed for pain relief.

Drugs

Beta-blockers are used to slow the heart rate, reduce the heart muscle's contractions, and lower blood pressure, thus reducing the workload on the heart.

Nitrates lower blood pressure by dilating the blood vessels. Most nitrates are used to relieve the symptoms of an angina attack once it has started or to prevent one in a situation that might precipitate it. These are taken as oral sprays or tablets placed under the tongue and offer relief within 5 minutes. People who suffer angina even when they are not exercising are often helped by longer-lasting forms of nitrate preparations, which are taken as tablets or absorbed slowly from a skin patch. Skin patches should be removed for eight hours before replacing to prevent a buildup of tolerance to the drug.

Calcium channel blockers also dilate the blood vessels by decreasing movement of calcium into the muscles surrounding the blood vessels. (Calcium is needed for the arterial muscles to contract.) They also reduce strain on the heart muscle by slowing the heart rate.

Surgery

For people whose angina is not sufficiently relieved by drugs or whose coronary arteries have been so narrowed by atherosclerosis that there is a high risk of heart attack, a more direct approach is needed. There are two surgical alternatives, which attempt to clear the blocked artery or bypass it.

Coronary angioplasty

In coronary angioplasty, a catheter with a small balloon at the tip is inserted into an artery in the arm or groin and threaded into the blocked coronary artery. When the catheter reaches the narrowed area, the balloon is then inflated for up to two minutes, pushing the walls of the artery apart. Catheters can also be fitted with lasers that vaporize blockages or with tiny cutters to shave off the atheroma from the artery walls. The fatty bits are then removed with a vacuum device.

Clearing out arteries
There are a number of different procedures using catheters to open arteries narrowed by plaques.

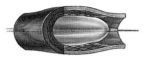

A balloon catheter is inserted into the artery and then inflated to push it open.

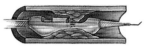

A catheter with a shaving device is used to shear plaque off the artery walls.

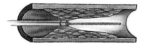

A laser beam may be emitted from the end of the catheter to vaporize the plaque.

Acupressure for angina
Apply pressure to these points during and after an angina attack.

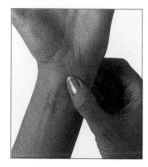

*PRESSURE POINT H 7
This point is on the wrist crease, just inside the small bone that aligns with the little finger.*

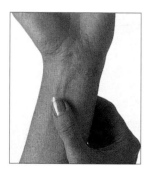

*PRESSURE POINT P 6
This point is located between the two tendons on the front of the wrist, two fingers away from the wrist crease.*

*CORONARY ARTERY BYPASS SURGERY
This may be done when attempts to clear blocked arteries have failed. In this illustration two of the coronary arteries have been bypassed.*

Coronary angioplasty and the new catheter techniques are generally simpler and safer procedures than coronary artery bypass grafting, but about a third of arteries cleared in this way become clogged again within a year, hence the necessity for making lifestyle changes to avoid this.

Coronary artery bypass

If blockages recur or if they are difficult to reach by catheter, your doctor may recommend surgery to bypass the affected area. In a coronary artery bypass procedure, a small length of vein, usually from the leg, is removed and grafted from the aorta to the coronary artery beyond the blockage to allow blood to flow to the heart muscle. Internal mammary and other arteries are often used. Usually two or three arteries are by-passed, but it can be as many as five.

During this operation, the heart is stopped and its functions and those of the lungs are temporarily taken over by a sophisticated piece of equipment called a cardiopulmonary bypass machine, commonly known as a heart-lung machine. Forty percent of those who have had this operation will have to have it again in 10 years.

Natural therapies

There are natural therapies that can be helpful in treating angina, but they must be used with your doctor's supervision. Treatments focus on reducing atherosclerosis (see page 108) and blood pressure (see page 124).

Acupuncture (see page 101) is widely used for angina in China. Acupressure, in which

hand or finger pressure is used instead of needles, can be just as effective. The symptoms of angina can be relieved by applying deep thumb pressure to H 7 and P 6 (see far left) for at least one minute. You might consult a practitioner of Chinese medicine and ask to be shown how to perform acupressure on yourself at home.

Angina can be reduced in severity by learning to relax and lower blood pressure. This can be achieved by autogenic training (see page 42) or biofeedback (see page 141), as well as meditation (see pages 36 and 104). Hypnosis can relieve the pain of angina and aid in relaxation.

HEART ATTACK (MYOCARDIAL INFARCTION)

If one or more coronary arteries becomes completely blocked, a heart attack (myocardial infarction) will result. During a heart attack an area of heart muscle dies from lack of blood and oxygen. The amount of damage to the heart depends on where the blockage occurs and how big an area of heart muscle dies.

A blockage can happen in two ways. Most commonly a blood clot, or thrombus (see page 125), suddenly obstructs the already narrowed artery, but occasionally atherosclerosis (see page 108) can be so severe that the artery simply clogs up completely.

Symptoms

The vast majority of heart attack victims suffer pain similar to that of angina, but it is more severe and longer lasting and does not cease with rest. In almost 70 percent of cases the pain radiates through the jaw and neck and down the left arm. Breathing can be difficult and labored and made worse by lying down. Nausea, dizziness, sweating, and belching up air are also common.

Once a heart-attack victim survives the early crisis, the chances of survival become increasingly better. Anyone who shows no signs of heart failure (see page 120) 48 hours after the onset of an attack, whose pulse is reasonably normal, and who does not have damage to the electrical pathways of the heart has a good chance of recovery.

Diagnosis

The principal tool doctors use to confirm a heart attack is an ECG (see page 91). However, changes to the heartbeat pattern

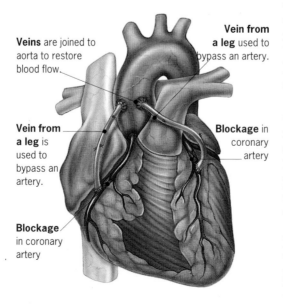

Veins are joined to aorta to restore blood flow.

Vein from a leg used to bypass an artery.

Vein from a leg is used to bypass an artery.

Blockage in coronary artery

Blockage in coronary artery

DID YOU KNOW?
Unlike angina, heart attacks rarely happen during vigorous exercise, such as on a squash court. It is more common for them to occur just afterward—in the changing room or during the drive home—probably because clots are less likely to form when blood flow is fast.

often do not appear until several hours after a heart attack starts and sometimes do not appear at all. Therefore, doctors generally rely on the patient's description of his or her symptoms and work on the assumption that a heart attack is taking place. The diagnosis can then be confirmed later.

Doctors can also monitor the patient's blood for enzymes that are released by the cells of damaged heart muscle. Among the easiest to measure is the enzyme creatine kinase (CK). The CK levels typically peak between 24 and 48 hours after a heart attack and remain raised for up to five days.

Treatment

Heart muscle can survive for only a few hours after its blood supply is cut off, so speed is vital in the treatment of someone who is suffering a heart attack. In this situation doctors have three priorities: to relieve pain, control abnormal heartbeat rhythms that develop, and prevent further damage to the heart muscle.

Intravenous injection of drugs from the opiate family, such as morphine (in most countries) and diamorphine (in the UK), better known as heroin, are frequently used to relieve pain. These medications work quickly and are very effective.

Many heart-attack sufferers develop dangerous abnormalities in their heart rhythm (see page 114), and these must be corrected quickly or they can prove fatal. Half of all heart-attack victims die from the most serious of these, ventricular fibrillation, in which the ventricles beat in such a fast and chaotic manner that hardly any blood is pumped around the body. The sufferer becomes unconscious, breathing stops, and death follows within minutes.

Certain drugs can be used to prevent this rhythm disturbance after a heart attack, while the use of a large electric shock (defibrillation) jolts the heart back into a normal rhythm and restores order. Clot-dissolving (thrombolytic) enzymes are given as soon as a heart attack is diagnosed—often on arrival at a hospital. Other treatment includes giving oxygen, if there is unstable angina, and nitroglycerine. Aspirin may also be given to prevent platelets from sticking together, as well as to treat pain (see page 114).

Depending on the patient's condition, he or she may be given beta-blockers (to reduce pain and make the heart beat more slowly); diuretics (if congestive heart failure occurs); and vasopressors (to raise blood pressure, or counter shock).

It is unlikely that one coronary artery will be completely blocked without the others also being clogged up to some extent. Either coronary angioplasty or a coronary artery bypass (see page 112) is sometimes needed to prevent another heart attack, but first the patient needs to be stabilized before invasive examinations and surgery are done.

Natural therapies

Recovering from a heart attack may involve medical procedures to unclog arteries, but you can adopt a number of measures that will go a long way toward preventing a heart attack and improving your chances of survival if you have already had one. Chapter 7 deals with recovery from a heart attack in more detail.

DURING A HEART ATTACK

The most obvious symptoms of a heart attack are crushing chest pain that lasts at least 20 minutes and a heaviness and tingling felt down the arms.

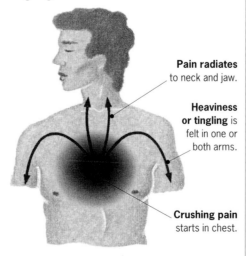

Pain radiates to neck and jaw.

Heaviness or tingling is felt in one or both arms.

Crushing pain starts in chest.

Caution with drugs

Heart drugs, many of which are dangerous if administered incorrectly, must always be used with caution. Make certain you understand all the instructions given on the label or by your doctor, and if you are unsure of anything, ask your doctor or pharmacist. Be sure to follow instructions exactly.

Discuss side effects with your doctor and contact him or her immediately if side effects become severe. Tell your doctor if symptoms persist because it may be possible or necessary to change your medication.

Always inform your doctor about any other medication you are taking, including the contraceptive pill and herbal remedies, as well as any chronic illnesses Also, let him or her know if you are pregnant or trying to conceive. Keep drugs in a cool, dry place, out of children's reach.

Herbal history
Many modern drugs have been extracted from natural herbs; one example is digitalis, which comes from foxglove. Digitalis causes the heart to beat more slowly, strengthens its contractions, and stimulates the kidneys to remove excess fluid from tissues. These properties were discovered in 1775 by William Withering, an English physician, and since that time digitalis has been widely prescribed for congestive heart failure. (The foxglove plant is highly poisonous and its extracts should be taken only under the supervision of a physician.)

Because atherosclerosis is the most common cause of coronary heart disease, it needs to be treated to prevent a heart attack (see page 108). Also, the control of hypertension is essential (see page 124).

A number of herbal remedies can help deal with the various factors that can lead to heart attack. These include bugleweed, motherwort, bromelain, mistletoe, and hawthorn (see page 102 for details about these and other helpful herbs). Ask a qualified herbalist for advice, and consult your doctor before you take any herbs.

HEART RATE AND RHYTHM DISORDERS

The heart's pacemaker, the sinoatrial node, controls the rate and rhythm of the heart by directing its electrical system (see page 20). There are two types of abnormal heart rhythms, or arrhythmias: those in which the heart beats too quickly, called tachycardia, and those in which the heart beats too slowly, known as bradycardia.

The most common cause of arrhythmia is coronary artery disease (see page 110). Inadequate blood supply to the heart disrupts the transmission of electrical signals around it. Arrhythmia also occurs during and after heart attacks (see page 112), when the heart's electrical pathways can be damaged, or as a result of congenital heart disorders (see page 106) or disorders of the thyroid gland (which produces hormones that stimulate the heart).

Symptoms
Both types of arrhythmias—tachycardia and bradycardia—can cause palpitations, dizziness, sudden fainting, and breathlessness because the heart beats less efficiently and less blood reaches the brain and lungs.

When the rhythm disturbance is severe, the person quickly becomes unconscious. If normal heart rhythm is not restored and the person resuscitated immediately, death follows in a few minutes.

Treatment
There are two main emergency methods of treating dangerous arrhythmias: jolting the heart back into a normal rhythm using a large electric shock, a procedure known as defibrillation, and/or the use of specialized anti-arrhythmic drugs (see page 113).

Patients who have mild symptoms do not require treatment. But in the case of an arrhythmia that causes severe symptoms,

ASPIRIN – THE WONDER DRUG?

In addition to its well-known properties of reducing fever and working as a painkiller and an anti-inflammatory, aspirin also acts as an antiplatelet, reducing the chances of a blood clot by preventing platelets from sticking together. For this last reason aspirin is often recommended by doctors for people who are at risk of a heart attack as well as those recovering from one or from a coronary bypass operation. The usual recommendation is 75 mg of aspirin a day.

Only low doses are required to produce an effect. This is the reason that "baby" aspirin is often recommended. The U.S. Doctors Aspirin Trial, which began in 1988, has shown a 44 percent decrease in the risk of heart attacks in people who have taken aspirin over five years.

Although aspirin reduces the chances of stroke caused by clots, at higher doses it increases the chance of stroke caused by bleeding (brain hemorrhage). However, at the low doses prescribed for heart disease there is no significant risk.

Aspirin can also cause severe stomach irritation and stomach bleeding in some cases. Specially coated, or enteric, pills can help sidestep these effects.

While doctors regard daily doses of aspirin as invaluable in treating some heart-disease patients, they do not recommend it in every case. People with a clotting disorder or a tendency to bleed, a stomach ulcer, an intolerance to aspirin, or asthma may be advised not to take it. Aspirin should be taken regularly only under medical supervision.

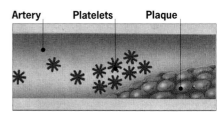

BEFORE TAKING ASPIRIN
When a cracked plaque in a blood vessel bleeds, platelets start to form clumps, thus leading to a clot.

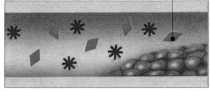

AFTER TAKING ASPIRIN
Aspirin reduces the stickiness of blood platelets so that they clump together less easily and a clot is less likely to form.

various long-term drugs may be prescribed, or a pacemaker, which enables the heart to beat normally, may be installed.

Pacemakers

A pacemaker is a small, battery-powered device. The battery, which is inserted under a flap of skin in the chest or stomach, is wired to an electrode implanted in the heart. The electrode sends out timed electrical impulses to make the heart contract and beat at a steady pace.

Pacemakers operate only when they sense the heart losing its rhythm. They are relatively easy to fit and their batteries last for 5 to 10 years before they need to be replaced with a small operation, which is usually carried out under local anesthetic.

People with pacemakers should avoid activities that might expose them to a strong electromagnetic field, such as working on a car engine while it is running. Contact sports or shooting with a rifle will interfere with the positioning of the device. Airport-monitoring equipment will not harm a pacemaker but the device itself may set off metal detectors.

Defibrillator

Patients with repeated tachycardia may have an automatic cardiac defibrillator implanted, which can return a rapidly beating heart to a normal rate and rhythm. The device is a small electric generator with three wires. It is implanted in the muscle of the abdomen, with an electrode positioned under the skin and the wires attached to the heart. It responds to an increase in heart rate with an electric shock that stops the heart for a split second, giving the sinoatrial node a chance to regain control.

Natural therapies

Arrhythmia needs to be treated medically, but some natural therapies can assist in relieving symptoms. Arrhythmia that results from a mineral deficiency may be treated with nutritional therapy, but only with the advice of a doctor or clinical dietitian. Magnesium maintains muscular contractions by balancing the effects of calcium (which makes muscles contract initially). Good sources of magnesium include nuts, soybeans and other legumes, and bran. Potassium, essential for slowing down the heart, is found in fruits and vegetables, with bananas being the best source.

RESTORING RHYTHM

The fitting of a pacemaker is done under local anesthetic. The pacemaker leads are threaded through a vein into the right ventricle, the right atrium, or both.

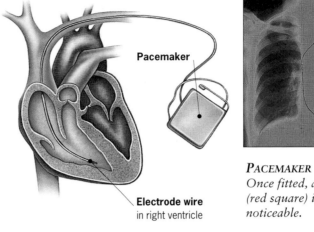

Pacemaker

Electrode wire in right ventricle

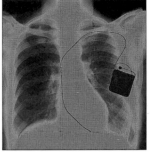

PACEMAKER IN PLACE
Once fitted, a pacemaker (red square) is scarcely noticeable.

Some herbs are recommended for irregularities in heart rhythm; these include bugleweed, night blooming cereus, lily-of-the-valley, and hawthorn berries. These are usually taken as teas. Consult an herbalist for the appropriate remedy and do not start taking herbs or stop taking medication without consulting your doctor.

Acupuncture and acupressure may help relieve palpitations by inducing relaxation. Stress management is essential for controlling arrhythmia. Meditation (see pages 36, 104), autogenic training (see page 42) and yoga (see page 104) can all be effective.

HEART-VALVE DISORDERS

The four valves of the heart ensure that blood travels in the right direction, and the heart's efficiency depends upon these valves working correctly (see pages 19–20). There are two types of valve disorders: The valves narrow and fail to open wide enough to allow sufficient blood through (stenotic); or the valves fail to close properly, allowing blood to flow backward (leaky, regurgitant, or incompetent).

Stenosis usually results from bacterial inflammation of the valve, an accumulation of calcium deposits caused by aging, or a valve abnormality that makes them more susceptible to calcium deposits. Leaky or regurgitant valves can be caused by heart disease, a bacterial infection known as endocarditis (see page 119), or rheumatic

ACUPRESSURE FOR ANXIETY: POINT H 3 Anxiety can bring on palpitations. Pressing this point at the end of the inner elbow crease when the elbow is bent will help you calm down.

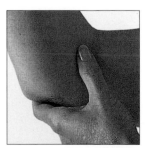

CARDIOPULMONARY RESUSCITATION (CPR)

CPR is an emergency first-aid procedure, used when the heart stops beating for more than a few seconds, to keep blood flowing to the brain, heart, and other organs and help a patient survive until medical help arrives. Carried out correctly, CPR can save lives, but rescuers must be properly trained. Broken ribs and internal bruising from poorly performed CPR may decrease the patient's chances of survival. Relatives or friends of anyone who is at high risk of a heart attack should learn CPR. The ABC formula forms the basis of CPR training. "A" is for airway, "B" is for breathing, and "C" is for compression.

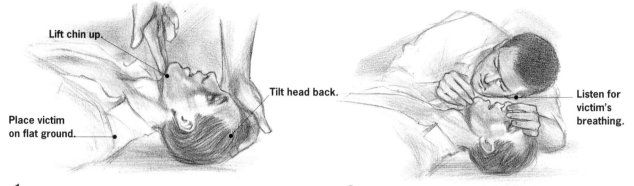

Lift chin up.

Tilt head back.

Place victim on flat ground.

Listen for victim's breathing.

1 *If the victim is unconscious and has no pulse, call for help immediately. Lay the victim on his or her back on a firm, flat surface. Kneel to the person's side. Clear the mouth of any objects such as food. To open the airways: put a hand on the victim's forehead and tilt it back. Place two fingers on the victim's lower jaw bone and lift it up to move the tongue away from the throat.*

2 *Check if the victim is breathing by listening for any breathing sounds, feeling for air movement on your cheek and ear and watching for chest movement. If the victim is not breathing, start mouth-to-mouth resuscitation.*

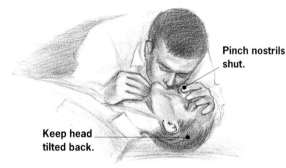

Pinch nostrils shut.

Keep head tilted back.

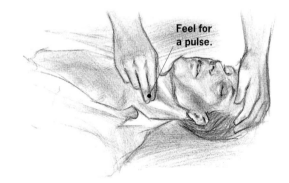

Feel for a pulse.

3 *Mouth-to-mouth: Keep the forehead tilted back and pinch the victim's nostrils shut. Open your mouth, take a deep breath and make a tight seal around the victim's mouth. Breathe slow breaths into the mouth—one breath every five seconds. Refill your lungs after each breath. The victim's chest should rise with each breath.*

4 *Feel for a pulse at the neck (carotid artery). If there is none, then compression is required.*

5 *Compression: Place the heel of your hand two fingers up from the bottom of the breastbone. Place your other hand on top of the first. Make sure your shoulders are directly over your hands and your elbows are straight and locked in order to use your own body weight for compression. Compress the chest smoothly and evenly, using the heel of your hand. Keep fingers off the victim's ribs. Apply enough force to depress the breastbone 4 to 5 cm (1½ to 2 in) at a rate of 80 compressions per minute. Between compressions, let the chest return to the normal position, but keep your hands in place on the chest. Count aloud. After 15 compressions, breathe into the victim's mouth twice. After four cycles of 15 compressions and two breaths, check again for a pulse and breathing. If there is none, continue the procedure until help arrives.*

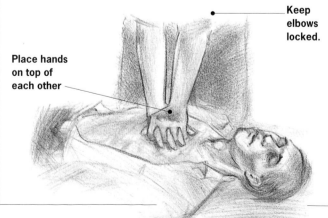

Keep elbows locked.

Place hands on top of each other

fever. Both types of valve disorder can also be congenital. The most common valve disorders involve the mitral and aortic valves on the left side of the heart.

Symptoms

The range of symptoms is wide. If the mitral valve between the left atrium and left ventricle becomes narrowed (stenotic), blood builds up in the atrium and goes back to the lungs. Blood vessels in the lungs, squeezed between this congestion on one side and blood being pumped in by the right ventricle on the other, begin to leak. Fluid enters the lung tissue and the lungs are unable to expand fully and take in adequate oxygen. The result is breathlessness, fatigue, and, in severe cases, congestive heart failure (see page 120). Additional possible complications are enlargement of the left atrium and development of arrhythmia (see page 114).

Mitral valve leakage (or regurgitation) is another common problem. In this case the cusps of the valve do not close properly and blood leaks back into the atrium when the left ventricle contracts. This reduces the amount of blood being pumped forward by the left ventricle, which has to work much harder to compensate. Symptoms may not

appear for years, but if the problem is not remedied, the left side of the heart is eventually weakened and permanently damaged by the strain. Symptoms develop that are similar to those of congestive heart failure, including shortness of breath, fatigue, weakness, swelling of the ankles, and palpitations.

Diagnosis

Doctors can glean quite a lot of information about how the valves are working by simply listening to the heart with a stethoscope (see page 20). If a doctor suspects that one or more valves are not functioning properly, several procedures can be used to establish what is going wrong and where. The most useful is echocardiography (see page 94), but X-rays and cardiac catheterization (see page 95) can also be used.

Treatment

Although treatment with diuretics, which encourage the loss of fluid from the body, can ease some of the symptoms, the best long-term solution is surgery to repair or replace the problematic valve.

Catheterization can be used to widen a narrowed valve in which there is limited blood flow. In a procedure known as

Rheumatic fever

Rheumatic heart disease was once a common outcome of rheumatic fever. Today this complication is rare because of antibiotics. Usually affecting children aged 5 to 15, rheumatic fever is a streptococcus (bacterial) infection. The symptoms include sore throat, chills, tender swollen glands, rapid heartbeat, joint pain, rash, and fatigue.

If it is not treated early with antibiotics, the infection can develop into an acute fever that lasts 10 to 14 days and attacks the heart valves. The valves become scarred, leading to malfunction, which may not be noticeable right away; in fact, it may not show up for 30 years. Some people have no problems or only mild discomfort for much of their lives. But eventually damaged heart valves will cause serious problems as the heart becomes less efficient.

INFECTION OF THE VALVES

Valve infections are most commonly caused by the bacteria *streptococcus viridans*. The infection starts as a sore throat and travels to the heart by way of

the blood. It is most likely to attack valves that are congenitally deformed or damaged by other diseases. A damaged valve may have to be surgically repaired.

STREPTOCOCCUS VIRIDANS
This micrograph shows the bacteria in their typical paired formation. The same bacteria may also be found in gut and tooth infections.

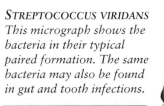
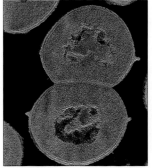

VALVE INFECTION
Bacteria may cause an inflammation of the valves.

Left atrium

Bacterial growth on the surface of the valves

Mitral valve

Aortic valve

Left ventricle

Endocardium lines the heart.

Prevent infection

Anyone with a heart valve problem should take extra care of their teeth and gums. Mouth infections can let bacteria into the bloodstream and cause further damage to the valves (a condition called infective endocarditis). Antibiotics should always be taken before dental treatment to prevent further risk of infection. Other serious infections, for example, in the urinary tract or the lungs, can also pose a risk, as can any kind of surgery.

DANDELION
The leaves and roots of the dandelion are effective diuretics that can help lower high blood pressure and reduce swelling in the legs.

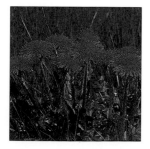

balloon valvuloplasty, a catheter fitted with a small balloon is inserted into an artery in the groin or arm and guided into the heart. Once inside the affected valve, the balloon is inflated, pushing the valve cusps apart. This procedure will have to be repeated if the cusps do not stay apart permanently.

Leaky or regurgitant valves can often be repaired, either by cutting out some sections of tissue to allow for a closer fit or by gathering in the surrounding tissue to push the valve cusps closer together. However, in many cases valves cannot be repaired and valve replacement is the only solution.

Replacement valves

There are two types of replacement valves: mechanical (made of metal and plastic) or biological (made from animal or donated human tissue, including pericardium from the patient's own heart or from someone who has died). Mechanical valves are tough and long-lasting but blood clots tend to form on their surfaces; patients fitted with mechanical replacement valves must have life-long treatment with anticoagulant drugs, which reduce the blood's normal tendency to clot. Biological valves do not cause this problem to such an extent but they are less durable; up to 50 percent of people must have the valve replaced within 10 years.

Natural therapies

Once valves are damaged, surgical repair or replacement is necessary. However, the symptoms of valve disease can be relieved by some natural measures. The most noticeable symptom is breathlessness, resulting from fluid buildup in the lungs. Herbal teas, such as dandelion and parsley, are mild diuretics that help reduce fluid buildup and relieve breathlessness. Unlike diuretic drugs, they do not leach the body of potassium. Check with your doctor before using these teas along with diuretic medication.

People with metal or plastic valves need anticoagulants. Herbalists recommend garlic, ginger, onion, and bromelain (from pineapple) as natural anticoagulants. Do not stop taking your anticoagulant medication without consulting your doctor.

HEART MUSCLE DISEASE

If the heart muscle becomes damaged, the heart loses its pumping power and, in severe cases, heart failure can follow. Disease of

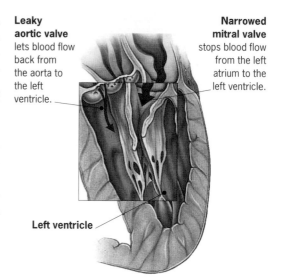

Leaky aortic valve lets blood flow back from the aorta to the left ventricle.

Narrowed mitral valve stops blood flow from the left atrium to the left ventricle.

Left ventricle

DISEASED VALVES
Valves may become narrowed or leaky, often as a result of infection. Some valves can be repaired, while others will have to be replaced.

the pericardium (the membrane surrounding the heart muscle) and the endocardium (the membrane lining the heart muscle) can also cause serious problems.

Disease of the heart muscle, called cardiomyopathy, has many causes. The muscle can be gradually weakened by a series of heart attacks; damaged by other conditions, such as coronary heart disease, high blood pressure, valve disease, neurological disorders, and blood disorders; or affected by alcoholism or a deficiency of nutrients such as thiamine (vitamin B_1).

There are three types of cardiomyopathy. Dilated cardiomyopathy occurs when the ventricle walls become weak and cannot pump efficiently. This condition may be caused by excessive alcohol, a viral infection, high blood pressure, or heart-valve defects. Hypertrophic cardiomyopathy results from thickening of the heart-wall muscles, which reduces the volume of the heart chambers and restricts the amount of blood pumped. Restrictive cardiomyopathy occurs when the heart's chambers do not fill properly, so blood goes backward into the veins. The causes are not well understood.

Inflammation of the heart muscle, called myocarditis, can occur as a result of viral or bacterial infections, chemicals, drugs, radiation, and immune system disorders. Most people will recover from myocarditis but some may suffer complications leading to heart failure or arrhythmia.

Alcohol and the heart

Excessive drinking can cause dilated cardiomyopathy. This occurs because alcoholics often do not eat properly, replacing food frequently with alcohol, and they develop deficiencies of nutrients, including vitamin B_1, B_2, B_3, B_6, folic acid, calcium, magnesium, and zinc. Also, alcohol itself and some of its chemical additives are toxic to the heart in large quantities.

If an alcoholic stops drinking before heart failure occurs, he or she may not suffer too much heart damage. However, heart muscle damage is irreversible, so once heart failure occurs, 50 percent of patients will die within a year and more than 75 percent of them will die within five years.

Giving up an alcohol addiction is not easy. However, once you have made the decision to do it, help is available. You can contact your local Alcoholics Anonymous (AA) organization, which will provide not only support but also encouragement and motivation through their self-help groups.

Some natural therapies, like acupuncture and hypnosis, can help overcome both the physical and psychological effects of withdrawal. Meditation can be used to strengthen willpower and combat withdrawal symptoms (see page 36). Yoga (see page 104) will keep you tranquil if you begin to feel depressed, anxious, or irritable during withdrawal. A naturopath (see page 122) or dietitian can help with advice on a healthy diet to replace the nutrients lost through excessive alcohol intake.

Pericarditis

If the pericardium, the tough protective bag or sac surrounding the heart, becomes infected by a virus or bacterium, an inflammation known as pericarditis can result. This causes pain that becomes worse with deep breathing or when the heart is beating rapidly. In some cases pericarditis causes the inner layer to produce too much lubricating fluid, which can compress the heart and reduce its ability to pump effectively. The pericardium may also thicken and become scarred, further restricting heart movement.

Endocarditis

Bacteria can also infect and cause inflammation in the lining of the heart chambers and valves, a condition known as endocarditis. A gum or tooth infection can bring this on, which is the reason that susceptible people must take antibiotics one hour before dental treatment and six hours after it.

Symptoms

Symptoms depend on the type of cardiomyopathy. Dilated cardiomyopathy causes palpitations, swollen ankles, breathlessness, and chest pain; hypertrophic cardiomyopathy causes breathlessness, chest pain, fatigue, and fainting; restrictive cardiomyopathy causes enlarged liver, swollen ankles, and fluid retention in the abdomen and lungs; myocarditis causes chest pain and shortness of breath; endocarditis produces the symptoms of valve disease (see page 117).

Treatment

Heart muscle infections caused by bacteria can be treated with antibiotics if they are detected promptly. Because there are often few specific symptoms until serious damage has occurred, early diagnosis is difficult. When the heart muscle becomes seriously damaged, however, heart transplantation is the only option.

Heart transplant

To qualify for this operation, individuals must be younger than 60 years and have a life expectancy of only two or three years. Potential candidates undergo a variety of

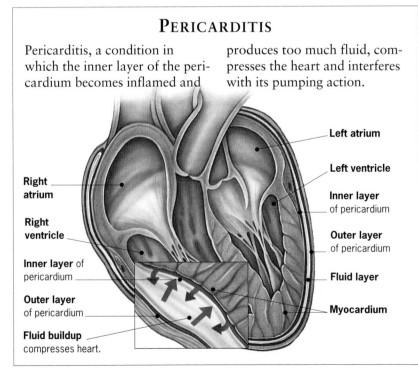

PERICARDITIS

Pericarditis, a condition in which the inner layer of the pericardium becomes inflamed and produces too much fluid, compresses the heart and interferes with its pumping action.

Right atrium

Right ventricle

Inner layer of pericardium

Outer layer of pericardium

Fluid buildup compresses heart.

Left atrium

Left ventricle

Inner layer of pericardium

Outer layer of pericardium

Fluid layer

Myocardium

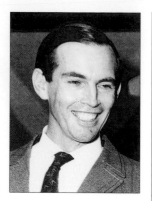

DR. CHRISTIAAN BARNARD
The world's first successful heart transplant from one human to another was carried out in 1967 by a South African surgeon, Christiaan Barnard.

tests to see if a heart transplant is appropriate. Contraindications, such as pulmonary hypertension, infection, a serious disease, drug or alcohol abuse, extreme obesity, or inability to stick to the program of medication, will rule them out. Tests will also be conducted to see if their immune system would reject the new heart.

If selected, the patient will be placed on a waiting list, and from that time until being called must stay within two to three hours of travel time to the hospital (a donor heart can survive for only 4 to 6 hours before the transplantation is completed). The donor of the heart must have the same blood group and tissue type as the recipient and have no sign of infection, but the donor's race and sex are of no importance. Although the heart size does not have to be the same, there cannot be too great a difference.

The transplant is a straightforward operation in skilled surgical hands. Patients are connected to the heart-lung machine and the old heart is removed by the surgeon who will make incisions in the atria, aorta, and pulmonary arteries and then connect the new heart to them.

After the surgery, patients must stay in the hospital for one to three weeks. To control rejection of the heart by the immune system they are given immunosuppressant drugs. These and other medications will have to be continued throughout life and will be adjusted to minimize side effects. Biopsies will be performed every week for the first six weeks following surgery to determine that the tissues are free from infection. This will continue biweekly for another six weeks, then monthly for three months, then quarterly and semi-annually. With a transplant, there is an 80 percent survival rate for one year and 60 percent after five years.

Natural therapies
Heart-muscle damage cannot be reversed, but some of the symptoms can be relieved. Such natural diuretics as dandelion tea can be taken to reduce fluid retention, and other herbs, like valerian, lemon balm, chamomile, and St. John's wort, can be used to promote relaxation.

CONGESTIVE HEART FAILURE
Congestive heart failure, also called simply heart failure, occurs when the heart can no longer pump enough blood to meet the

body's demands. The process is gradual and can often take many years. Any damage to the pumping capacity of the heart caused by high blood pressure, coronary heart disease, heart attack, rhythm disorders, or valve defects or disease can lead to heart failure.

Once heart failure has begun, it gets progressively worse. The heart compensates for failing to meet the body's demands for blood by pumping faster and harder. The arteries contract, making the already struggling heart's task of pumping blood around the body much more difficult. Also, pressure builds in the veins because the heart is not able to pump blood efficiently through the arteries. These effects make the heart grow progressively weaker.

Meanwhile, the poor circulation of blood to the kidneys means they cannot function properly or excrete enough sodium in the urine. Levels of sodium rise, causing water retention in the body and a general buildup of fluid in the body tissues, which puts further pressure on the heart.

Symptoms
Symptoms of heart failure include shortness of breath, even at rest, which becomes worse when lying down because of a buildup of fluid in the lungs; fatigue during exercise; and swelling of the legs, feet, hands, and sometimes trunk of the body. Heart failure can be mild or severe, but it is often referred to as congestive because of the filling of the lungs and tissues with fluid.

Left or right heart failure
Doctors often refer to left-heart failure or right-heart failure, depending on which side of the heart is most affected. The job of the left atrium and ventricle is to take oxygenated blood from the lungs and pump it around the body. Therefore, left-heart failure results in fluid accumulating in the lungs. This means that breathlessness is the most important symptom.

The job of the right atrium and ventricle is to collect deoxygenated blood returning from the body and pump it to the lungs. During right-heart failure, the blood flow is also decreased, but in this case, the fluid that accumulates produces swelling in the legs, stomach, and liver.

Both left- and right-heart failure ultimately result in less blood being pumped to the body, causing general fatigue.

Diagnosis

Doctors establish a preliminary diagnosis of heart failure from a physical examination and the patient's symptoms, and then confirm this using X-ray and echocardiography examinations (see page 94).

Treatment

Rest can play an important role in the treatment of heart failure. If the patient is very elderly or is content with an inactive lifestyle, there may be no point in further treatment because heart failure generally progresses slowly and the symptoms are greatly improved by rest.

There are several other ways to minimize the discomfort of heart failure. Lose weight, if necessary (see page 51); reduce the amount of salt in your diet (see page 51); limit your fluid intake to two liters (two quarts) a day, except during hot weather or when you are suffering from an illness, diarrhea, or fever. Additional recommendations include drinking alcohol only in moderate amounts or not at all; not smoking at all; and trying to do some regular mild exercise, such as walking for 20 minutes daily. For this last, take care not to overstrain yourself.

Drugs

The symptoms of heart failure can be relieved by long-term treatment with drugs, like digitalis, which strengthen and regulate the heart's pumping action; diuretics, which reduce the amount of fluid in the body; and vasodilators, such as ACE (angiotensin-converting enzyme) inhibitors, which widen the constricted blood vessels and thus reduce the pressure against which the heart has to pump, easing its workload.

Sluggish blood circulation means that people suffering from heart failure are more at risk for the formation of blood clots (thrombus), which can block vital arteries. They are therefore often given anticoagulant therapy, which helps to prevent clotting. All grades of heart failure can usually be controlled with diuretics or ACE inhibitors and by reducing the amount of salt in the diet. As a result of advances in drug therapy, the outlook for heart-failure patients has greatly improved. However, while the majority of cases can be treated with one or more of the drugs mentioned above, if heart failure becomes severe, a heart transplant may be the only hope (see page 119).

Natural therapies

There are no natural therapies that will restore a failed heart, but there are some measures that can help relieve symptoms. Herbal diuretic teas—dandelion or parsley, for instance—can be taken to reduce fluid retention. Check with your doctor first to be sure they will not conflict with a prescribed diuretic. You can also increase your intake of onion, garlic, and ginger, which have anticoagulant effects.

Acupressure, massage, and hydrotherapy can help relieve swelling in the legs and improve the circulation.

CONGESTIVE HEART FAILURE

Heart failure results in a build-up of blood in the veins and pushing of fluid into the tissues.

The symptoms depend on whether the left or right side of the heart has failed.

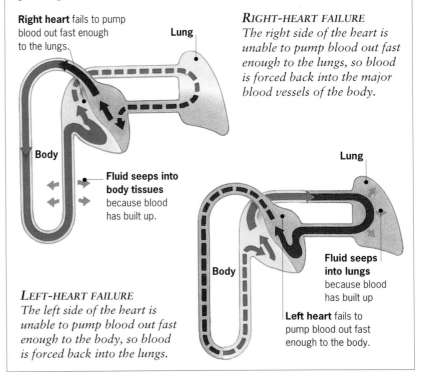

Right heart fails to pump blood out fast enough to the lungs.

Lung

Body

Fluid seeps into body tissues because blood has built up.

RIGHT-HEART FAILURE
The right side of the heart is unable to pump blood out fast enough to the lungs, so blood is forced back into the major blood vessels of the body.

Lung

Fluid seeps into lungs because blood has built up

Body

Left heart fails to pump blood out fast enough to the body.

LEFT-HEART FAILURE
The left side of the heart is unable to pump blood out fast enough to the body, so blood is forced back into the lungs.

The Naturopath

Dealing with heart disorders requires attention to rest, exercise, nutritional needs, and stress management. A naturopath will give advice on these matters, based on an individual's symptoms.

Origins

The idea of naturopathic medicine began with Hippocrates over two millennia ago. He believed that attention to diet, rest, and exercise was the key to health. In Europe during the 1800s a kind of naturopathy that focused on hydrotherapy, as well as dietary measures, was developed by therapists such as Vincent Preissnitz. An Austrian priest, Father Sebastian Kneipp (1821–1897), originated a special water cure, which was brought to the United States by one of his followers, Benedict Lust, at the turn of the century. Lust established the first school of naturopathy in New York.

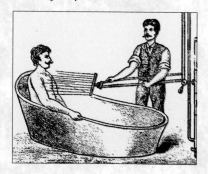

WATER CURES
This variable pressure shower, used to stimulate the circulation, was a popular practice of early hydrotherapy.

Naturopaths have the skills to advise and guide patients with heart disease toward a program that will suit their individual needs and help rebuild their health, so they can lead a longer and more fulfilling life.

What is naturopathy?
Naturopathic medicine is a system of health care that helps to mobilize and support the body's self-healing processes. A naturopath uses various natural approaches rather than one specific therapy. The emphasis is always on measures that are in harmony with nature and are tailored to the individual's needs. The naturopath's objective is to help patients take more responsibility for their own well-being and develop their potential for better health.

What happens at the consultation?
At an initial consultation, a naturopath will question you about your health problems and how they are affected by the food you eat, your work, exercise and other aspects of your lifestyle, even the weather.

Previous illnesses and injuries, which may have a bearing on the way your body deals with a present disorder, will also be noted. An illness like rheumatic fever in childhood, for example, may have caused a weakness in the heart valves that is not evident until later in life, when weakening of the heart makes it more difficult to compensate for it.

The naturopath will carry out a complete examination, including measuring your pulse rate and blood pressure, listening to your heart and lungs, inspecting your skin, eyes, and other areas, and ordering standard blood and urine analyses.

The practitioner will then discuss possible treatments with you, emphasizing measures you can carry out yourself. Because naturopathy is holistic in its approach, he or she will help you seek the possible cause of any conditions you have.

What sort of treatments do naturopaths prescribe?
A naturopath will take into account your doctor's diagnosis and treatment of your heart problem and will then decide what you can do in the way of diet, exercise, and other measures to cope more effectively and improve the health of your heart.

A naturopath will also make recommendations on ways you can reduce physical and emotional stress on your heart and strengthen and sustain its function. This may take the form of herbal and/or nutritional supplements or a diet of raw fruit and vegetable juices only. You will be given guidelines for rest and relaxation and appropriate exercises. Special baths, compresses, or other forms of hydrotherapy may be advised to help improve circulation.

Naturopaths generally recommend things you can do at home, but certain therapies, such as massage or acupuncture, must be done in the office. These will improve the self-healing processes in your body but not conflict with any conventional medical treatment you are receiving.

How does the naturopath decide which treatments to give?

The naturopath's consultation and examination is intended to reach a diagnosis of your specific condition, as well as an assessment of how it relates to your overall health and vitality. Some calculations using your blood pressure and pulse rate, for example, will give the practitioner a useful guide to the amount of tension in your circulatory system. If it is low, this may indicate weakness and loss of vitality, and a naturopath might suggest a warming and energy-producing diet. High tension suggests more pressure and congestion in the body, and to improve this condition, you may be advised to eat more raw fruits and vegetables.

The naturopath will also decide whether you need stress-relieving instruction or if acupuncture or massage may benefit you.

What recommendations does a naturopath make for heart disease?

Your naturopath will first make sure that you have a good basic diet. A healthy diet helps to detoxify the body and provides antioxidant nutrients (see page 58), which protect cells against damage.

Naturopaths can also give advice on special diet regimens to improve specific problems associated with heart trouble. To relieve fluid retention caused by circulatory problems, a naturopath might suggest following a strict diet for a few days, including cutting out salt and taking natural diuretics. (Any special diet should be followed only under the supervision of a naturopath and you should check with your doctor before commencing it.)

What sort of exercise will a naturopath suggest for the heart?

There are many forms of exercise that can be beneficial for the heart such as walking, swimming, gardening, yoga, and t'ai chi. The naturopath will tailor activity to the individual's needs.

Do naturopaths prescribe nutritional supplements for heart patients?

While placing an emphasis on a balanced whole-food diet, most naturopaths recognize the need for extra antioxidant nutrients in anyone who has heart disease. Beta carotene (vitamin A) and vitamins C and E may all be indicated in appropriate doses in addition to minerals, such as magnesium, for sufferers of angina and other disorders in which blood vessels are constricted. Appropriate forms and dosages of supplements must be determined by a practitioner.

Will naturopathic treatment conflict with my doctor's advice?

Naturopathy is directed at improving the self-healing processes in your body, and it will usually not conflict with conventional medical treatment. Many doctors now recognize the important complementary role that naturopathy can play in total health care and will refer patients to qualified practitioners. You do not need a medical referral to seek the advice of a naturopath, but if you are on any kind of medication, you should consult your doctor before beginning any naturopathic treatment.

Where can I find a naturopath?

In the United States naturopaths train at one of two colleges of naturopathic medicine. The American Association of Naturopathic Physicians in Seattle, Washington, lists qualified practitioners. People in Canada can contact the Canadian Naturopathic Association for a list.

Most naturopaths work in private practice, but some hold posts in residential naturopathic clinics that have spa baths and other facilities.

WHAT YOU CAN DO AT HOME

Good quality sleep is essential for your body to repair damaged tissues, particularly those affected by a heart attack. You can improve your sleep without resorting to any medication with a simple hydrotherapy method in your own bathroom.

Just before going to bed, sponge or spray your lower legs (below the knees) with cold water for one or two minutes and dry them off. When you climb into bed, your feet will be warm and sleep will generally follow easily. You can repeat the process if you are restless during the night.

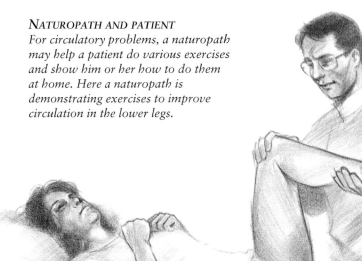

NATUROPATH AND PATIENT
For circulatory problems, a naturopath may help a patient do various exercises and show him or her how to do them at home. Here a naturopath is demonstrating exercises to improve circulation in the lower legs.

CIRCULATORY DISORDERS

The health of your arteries and veins can be impaired by a variety of factors, and the resulting damage may lead to life-threatening conditions such as stroke.

Blockages or degeneration can occur in any of the blood vessels in the body, with various effects.

HYPERTENSION

Each time the heart beats it creates a wave of pressure that pushes blood along the arteries and veins of the body. Hypertension is blood pressure that stays abnormally high over a prolonged period, even when resting.

About 50 million Americans suffer from hypertension. Among Canadians, 25 percent of men and 18 percent of women are afflicted. Because in its early stages, the condition is symptomless, many people don't realize they have this life-threatening disease.

Like any pumping system, the body's circulation can work efficiently only within a certain range of pressure. If the pressure is too low, not enough blood reaches vital organs, including the brain. If it is too high for a prolonged period, the extra pressure damages the heart and blood vessels and wreaks havoc on the inside walls of arteries, making the development of atherosclerosis more likely. Hypertension also doubles the risk of heart attack, increases the risk of stroke fourfold, and causes kidney failure.

Causes

Hypertension has a specific cause in about 10 percent of cases. Among the possibilities are obesity; heart disorders; kidney problems; a disorder of the adrenal glands, which produce hormones that help regulate blood pressure; thyroid problems; and the side effects of some drugs—oral contraceptives, for instance, and medications used for treating ulcers and arthritis. In addition, blood pressure tends to rise as people grow older and their arteries and other blood vessels become less flexible. The middle-aged and elderly are especially at risk and should have their blood pressure checked once a year. In the majority of cases, however, no specific cause can be found; doctors refer to this condition as essential hypertension.

Symptoms

Hypertension rarely causes any symptoms and can therefore silently undermine an individual's health over a number of years. Such signs as dizziness, headache, blurred vision, and tiredness arise only when blood pressure is extremely high. Normally, symptoms do not appear until the body has been damaged by prolonged high blood pressure.

Treatment

Many people with hypertension can lower their blood pressure into the healthy range through a few simple lifestyle changes: a low-fat diet, more exercise, stress reduction, and giving up smoking. Those who find such changes difficult and whose condition is persistent, severe, and damaging to organs like the heart and kidneys will require medication, sometimes for life.

Drugs

Drugs commonly prescribed for persistent hypertension include beta-blockers, ACE (angiotension converting enzyme) inhibitors, diuretics—to eliminate excess fluid, which increases blood pressure—and vasodilators. As with all drugs, antihypertensives, as they are known, have potential side effects, and different medications will be better suited to different individuals. Generally, however, the side effects caused by antihypertensives tend to be mild and usually do not interfere with a normal, active life.

FOCUS ON HYPERTENSION
Blood vessels in the eye are quickly affected by high blood pressure, and blurred vision may result. Examination of the eyes can be a useful way to diagnose hypertension because the doctor will see burst blood vessels.

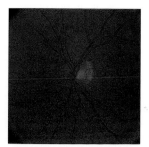

Natural therapies

There is no doubt that changes in lifestyle and diet, plus other natural approaches, can lower hypertension, but they can also reduce the need for antihypertensives, so your doctor must be informed of methods you are using and monitor your progress.

Naturopaths often recommend a diet of mineral-rich foods for reducing high blood pressure. This includes calcium (dairy products, sesame seeds, spinach and broccoli), magnesium (nuts, beans, dark green leafy vegetables and seafood) and potassium (fish, bananas, potatoes, avocados, tomatoes, apricots, and peaches).

Herbalists prescribe mild diuretics such as lily- of-the-valley and dandelion and parsley to decrease fluid retention. Herbs infusions that can be taken in place of regular tea and coffee include chamomile and valerian.

Acupuncture and acupressure (see page 101) can help to reduce high blood pressure, but should not replace medication. Try pressure point LI 4 as shown (right).

Biofeedback (see page 141) has been proven in many studies to be effective in enabling an individual to reduce his or her own blood pressure by becoming aware of how the body reacts to various factors.

For the reduction of stress, aromatherapists suggest adding a few drops of lavender oil to a warm bath. An aromatherapy massage using oils specific to your condition can also be therapeutic.

Homeopathy can be successful in treating high blood pressure, but it is essential to consult a trained therapist.

Yoga (see page 104) has been proven to reduce stress and high blood pressure. In a study of 3,000 hypertensive people done in 1984, some 84 percent of them improved.

THROMBOSIS AND EMBOLISM

Blood clotting is a natural safety mechanism of the body that prevents excessive bleeding, but sometimes the clots themselves can cause problems.

Thrombosis

A thrombus is a blood clot that forms inside a blood vessel. This may be caused by atherosclerosis (see page 108), as the fatty deposits become hard and then crack and bleed. Blood clots form and may grow large enough to block the blood vessel. If the vessel is a coronary artery, this can cause a heart attack; if it is a blood vessel supplying the brain, the result can be a stroke.

A deep-vein thrombosis is a blood clot in a deep vein of the leg or pelvis that causes inflammation. The thrombus results from an injury to the vein wall or stagnation of

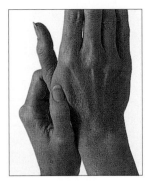

ACUPRESSURE POINT LI 4 FOR HYPERTENSION This point is at the bottom of the crease formed by pressing the thumb and index finger together. Apply firm pressure for a few minutes every day.

YOGA FOR HYPERTENSION

The following routine is good for relieving tension and is safe to do. To learn additional relaxing poses, it is advisable to join a yoga class, in which an instructor can teach you exercises specific to your health needs. You can then practice them at home when you know how to do them correctly.

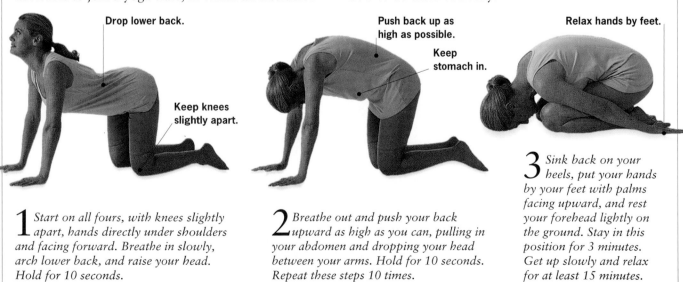

Drop lower back.

Keep knees slightly apart.

Push back up as high as possible.

Keep stomach in.

Relax hands by feet.

1 *Start on all fours, with knees slightly apart, hands directly under shoulders and facing forward. Breathe in slowly, arch lower back, and raise your head. Hold for 10 seconds.*

2 *Breathe out and push your back upward as high as you can, pulling in your abdomen and dropping your head between your arms. Hold for 10 seconds. Repeat these steps 10 times.*

3 *Sink back on your heels, put your hands by your feet with palms facing upward, and rest your forehead lightly on the ground. Stay in this position for 3 minutes. Get up slowly and relax for at least 15 minutes.*

Blood clots

Blood clots can form in both arteries and veins and block the blood supply to an organ. A blood clot can also travel from one place in the body to another.

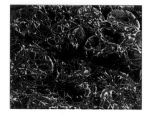

BLOOD CLOT
This thrombus, magnified 2,200 times, is composed of red blood cells trapped in a network of fibrin (yellow) strands. A thrombus usually forms when blood flow is blocked in an artery.

CORONARY THROMBOSIS
This thrombus (the clump of red, lower center) is seen protruding from an arterial entrance to a chamber of the heart. It is likely to cause a heart attack.

the blood flow while a person is confined to bed during a long illness or after surgery. For this reason hospital patients are encouraged to get out of bed as soon as possible, or they are given a routine of leg exercises and physiotherapy sessions. Many also have to wear elastic stockings, which temporarily increase the blood pressure in the legs and prevent clots from forming. Sometimes anticoagulant drugs are also prescribed.

Embolism

Part or all of a thrombus that breaks off and is carried in the blood to other areas is called an embolus, and it causes an embolism (blockage). Some other causes of blockage include atheromas, fat globules, cancer tumors, air bubbles, and amniotic fluid from the uterus in pregnancy. These may travel in the bloodstream until they lodge in and block a narrower vessel.

Pulmonary embolism occurs when a deep-vein thrombus breaks off and is carried to the pulmonary artery that feeds the lungs. The embolus can block the vessel, cutting off some or all of the blood supply to the lungs, often with fatal consequences.

Virtually any area of the body can be affected by an embolism. They commonly occur where arteries branch and block one or both branches. The possible consequences include stroke, caused by a cerebral embolism; gangrene, caused by an embolus blocking an artery in the leg; and reduction in oxygenated blood, caused by a pulmonary (lung) embolism that has traveled from a deep vein.

Symptoms

The symptoms of thrombosis and embolism depend on where and how severe the blockage is. Any obstruction to an artery reduces the amount of fresh oxygenated blood it can

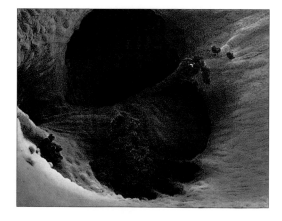

supply. If the blockage is serious enough, the organ or area of the body that is supplied by the artery will begin to die. If it is an area of heart muscle, a heart attack can ensue. If it is part of the brain, a stroke may be the result. These are sudden events, and normally there is no warning. However, if the area affected is distant from the heart—in an arm, leg, fingers, or toes—the area may become cold, white, and painful. In severe cases, skin and muscle may die and become gangrenous and the affected part may have to be amputated.

Diagnosis

When an artery becomes blocked, blood flow and therefore blood pressure downstream of the obstruction is reduced. This fact is often used by doctors to investigate a suspected thrombosis or embolism. First, blood pressure is measured in an arm to gain information about the overall blood flow. Then, blood pressure is measured in the place where a blockage is suspected—in one of the legs, for example—and compared with that in the arm.

Blood pressure measurement can also be used to test for blockages in the carotid arteries in the neck, which supply the brain. Small branches of these arteries supply the eyes, and measuring blood pressure there provides valuable information. This is done using tiny devices that sit on the front of the eyes like contact lenses.

Often these simple tests can give doctors enough information to locate and treat the blockage, but sometimes more detailed investigation, such as angiography, is needed (see page 98), to see the blood flow and the exact position of the blockage.

Treatment

Thrombosis and embolism can be treated with clot-dissolving (thrombolytic) drugs. These are piped directly to the affected area using a catheter. People who have had a thrombus or embolism may be prescribed anticoagulant drugs for the long term to prevent a recurrence.

However, if these drugs do not work, an operation known as an embolectomy may be necessary. A catheter is inserted into the artery and then pushed gently through the blockage. A tiny balloon at the end of the catheter is inflated. The catheter and balloon are carefully withdrawn, bringing the clot, or

EXERCISE FOR THROMBOSIS

A blood clot may occur as a result of atherosclerosis. It is also common in bedridden patients due to lack of activity.

The following exercises can be done by inactive people to improve circulation in the legs and prevent clots from forming.

ANKLE FLEXING
Sit on a chair with shoes off. Bend ankle forward and backward and circle it around. Repeat with the other ankle.

Relax upper body.

Flex ankle in all directions.

KNEE BENDS
Holding onto a chair for balance, bend leg backward at the knee. Repeat 10 times with each leg at least once a day.

Hold onto a chair for balance.

Raise foot as high as it goes.

Keep moving
The more you sit in one place, the more you increase your chances of developing a blood clot. This is particularly true during extended travel by airplane. To avoid this, wear loose clothing and roomy shoes. Take a walk around the plane once an hour and stretch your legs periodically when seated.

whatever has caused the obstruction, with it. In severe cases it may be necessary to bypass the blocked artery (see page 112) by removing a vein from another part of the body and grafting it to the artery on either side of the blockage to bypass the obstruction.

Natural therapies
Natural therapies can help decrease the chance of blood clots forming. Naturopaths advise eating onions, garlic, ginger, and bromelain (in pineapple) for preventing clots. Lecithin, a type of fat, decreases the stickiness of blood platelets, thus reducing the risk of clotting. Some natural therapists advise lecithin supplements, but dietary sources, such as soybeans, are adequate.

The antioxidant vitamins A, C, and E (see page 59) are recommended. Some therapists suggest taking supplements, but eating at least five servings a day of fruits and vegetables should give you sufficient quantities of A and C. Whole grains and nuts provide E.

The pain of blood clots can often be relieved by the use of herbal lotions, compresses, and poultices. Arnica and comfrey are commonly used for this purpose.

STROKE
A stroke is a brain injury that results from an interruption in the blood supply. This occurs when an artery becomes blocked by a thrombus or an embolism or because a blood vessel in the brain ruptures. The affected area of brain tissue dies.

Strokes that are caused by a thrombosis or embolism are more common in middle-aged or elderly people, whose arteries may have become clogged by atherosclerosis over the years. Strokes caused by the sudden rupture of blood vessels in the brain (cerebral hemorrhage) also affect the young.

Symptoms
A stroke that is caused by an embolism is a sudden event and there is no warning. If, however, the problem is due to clotting in the main artery that runs up the neck and supplies the brain (known as the carotid artery), there may be some warning signs, including bouts of weakness; confusion and difficulties with speech; and tingling or clumsiness in a limb. If the stroke is caused by the rupture of a blood vessel, a severe headache will precede it.

The effects of a stroke vary depending on the location of the blockage, as well as its extent. In a cerebral thrombosis, a blood clot forms within the walls of a cerebral blood vessel, causing an obstruction to blood flow. Permanent brain damage will result if the blood supply is completely stopped or if it is reduced to less than a quarter of its normal level.

In the case of a cerebral embolism, a blood clot or other matter (see page 126) that has traveled to the brain from another part of the body—an artery in the neck, for example—obstructs a cerebral artery. Such clots most often lodge in the left middle cerebral artery, where they cause weakness or paralysis in the right side of the body and, in addition, can affect memory, speech, and personality.

If the stroke occurs in the right side of the brain, the left side of the body will be affected and, in addition to paralysis, there may be speech, calculation, and sensation difficulties and a loss of the ability to recognize pictures, objects, and colors. There may also be unsteadiness, dizziness, and nausea.

Mild strokes last from a few minutes to less than a day and cause minor symptoms, such as dizziness, speech difficulties, vision problems, and nausea. These are usually warning signs that a more serious stroke is imminent; prompt treatment may prevent permanent damage from occurring. More serious strokes have more critical consequences, including paralysis, loss of speech and vision, loss of control over bodily functions, and mental confusion.

Diagnosis

Techniques used to confirm the diagnosis of a stroke include angiography and computed tomography, also known as a CAT or CT scan (see page 95), which uses X-rays linked to a computer to produce a cross-sectional image of the head and brain, and magnetic resonance imaging, or MRI (see page 95), which does much the same thing using magnetic fields and radio waves.

Treatment

Anticoagulant drugs are often given to prevent another stroke, and some ruptures, blood clots, and embolisms can be dealt with by surgery. (Anticoagulants are not given in hemorrhagic strokes.) But generally the treatment centers on rehabilitation.

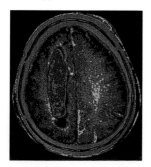

BRAIN HEMORRHAGE
This CT scan of the brain of a stroke patient shows a hemorrhage (the orange oval shape on the left) caused by the rupture of blood vessels resulting from hypertension.

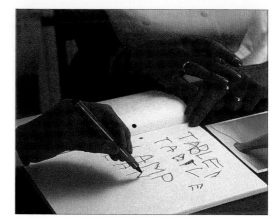

STROKE REHABILITATION
This patient had a stroke in the left side of her brain and so she can no longer write with her right hand. In this picture, she is being taught to write with her left hand.

Rehabilitation

Nursing care and intensive physiotherapy aim to restore as much of an affected person's former abilities as possible. For maximum recovery, rehabilitation should start immediately after a stroke

First, a patient is taught balance, which is commonly affected by a stroke. Then, gentle supervised exercise begins, usually with walking practice. It may take one to six months for the patient to learn to walk unaided. Swimming with the assistance of a trained therapist is invaluable for improving mobility and strength, both of which are often impaired after a stroke.

Therapy is often needed also for speech and vision, which may be partially or even fully recovered if rehabilitation treatment starts early with qualified professionals.

Natural therapies

Natural therapies can help in recovering from an embolic stroke, but should be undertaken only with your doctor's advice. A healthy diet, including anticoagulant foods (onion, garlic, and ginger) can not only aid recovery but also help to prevent another stroke. Naturopaths suggest that stroke patients take supplements of vitamins E and C, evening primrose oil, lecithin, and fish oils.

A few herbs can help improve circulation in stroke patients. They include rosemary, mistletoe, and cayenne. Pour a cup of boiling water over 2 teaspoons of dried herb and steep for 15 minutes. Drink the beverage hot three times a day.

Homeopaths (see page 103) often prescribe *Arnica 200c* to be taken as soon as possible after a stroke. To dissolve clots, *Arnica 6c* and *Kali mur 6x* should be taken twice a day for one month.

Acupuncture (see page 101) can help to stimulate circulation as well as to promote relaxation, both of which are important for the prevention of another stroke.

Massage (see page 100) helps to stimulate the circulation and prepare a stroke patient for exercise sessions. Aromatherapy oils can be chosen specifically for this purpose.

ANEURYSM

An aneurysm is a ballooning of an artery wall, usually resulting from damage to the wall caused by atherosclerosis or hypertension. It may also be congenital.

Small ones, called berry aneurysms, are commonly found in the brain arteries. Warning signs of their existence include a drooping eyelid, dilated pupils, and double vision, but they can exist for years and be symptom free. A ruptured brain aneurysm causes serious bleeding, usually felt as a severe headache, and a stroke.

Aneurysms are also found in the aorta. The swelling may eventually split the wall of the aorta and will be felt as a large lump in the abdomen. Aneurysms can cause many problems it they burst; press on organs, nerves, or blood vessels; or form a clot.

AORTIC ANEURYSM
Aneurysms can occur in the aorta and may displace organs and blood vessels. As shown here, blood flow to and from the left kidney is being blocked by an aneurysm.

Kidney displaced by aneurysm

Ureter displaced by aneurysm

Renal vein displaced by aneurysm

Aneurysm in aorta

Diagnosis
Brain aneurysms are most often diagnosed with a CT scan (see page 95). Aneurysms elsewhere can be seen on X-rays and ultrasound scans (see page 94).

Treatment
Aneurysms cannot be reversed, but they can sometimes be prevented from getting larger by a reduction in blood pressure. Usually aneurysms, particularly aortic aneurysms, are removed by surgery before they rupture to avoid serious damage. Often, part of the wall of the aorta must be replaced with some artificial tubing.

Natural therapies
Once an aneurysm is formed there is no alternative to surgery for treating it. However, a healthy cholesterol and blood pressure level can go a long way toward preventing aneurysms (see atherosclerosis, page 108, and hypertension, page 124).

INTERMITTENT CLAUDICATION
This is a pain that occurs during walking or other exercise in the thigh and calf muscles, buttocks, or arch of the foot. It is caused by a restriction in the blood supply to the leg, usually resulting from atherosclerosis (a buildup of fatty deposits) in the leg arteries. It is particularly common in people who smoke. Exercise increases the muscles' demand for glucose and oxygen, which cannot be met because of the blockage in the blood supply, resulting in cramps.

Intermittent claudication may occur in just one or both legs. If left untreated, blood clots may form and cut off the blood supply to the muscles. Gangrene will result and amputation will be necessary.

Treatment
The most important action is to stop smoking. Regular exercise will improve the blood supply to the legs. Pain felt during exercise will stop during rest.

Drugs may be given to dilate the arteries and reduce blood clotting. These will not stop progression of the condition, however, without commensurate changes in a smoking habit, diet, and exercise. Dietary changes include reducing saturated fats.

In severe cases, bypass surgery (see page 112) or balloon angioplasty (see page 111) may be performed to clear blocked arteries.

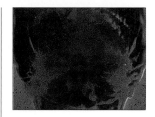

BRAIN ANEURYSM
This angiogram shows a "berry" aneurysm (the round orange nodule), which occurs where an artery branches in the brain. It is caused by a congenital defect and can burst as a result of high blood pressure.

Which kind of cramp?
Everyone is bound to suffer leg cramps at some point, so it is important to know which ones are simply due to overworked or unfit muscles and which result from arterial disease. Those caused by the former are constant, usually go away with stretching or massage, and do not recur on a regular basis. Cramps caused by arterial disease are intermittent, usually occur with any exercise, even just walking, and stop when you rest. If you are experiencing leg cramps even when doing mild exercise, seek the advice of your doctor.

129

SELF-HELP FOR VARICOSE VEINS

To prevent varicose veins, keep your weight within normal limits, avoid standing for long periods of time, exercise regularly, and wear flat shoes. If you already have varicose veins, try these measures to relieve them.

▶ *Wear support stockings.*

▶ *Start an exercise program—walking and swimming are best.*

▶ *When sitting or lying down, elevate your legs above hip level.*

▶ *If a vein bursts and bleeds, bandage it tightly and keep the leg raised until the bleeding stops. Consult your doctor as soon as possible.*

Natural therapies

Because intermittent claudication is usually caused by atherosclerosis, treatment is directed at this disorder (see page 108). Naturopaths recommend walking for one hour daily and taking vitamin E supplements (consult a naturopath for amounts). Also, eat foods that are rich in magnesium, such as nuts, beans, peas, and whole-grain cereals.

The homeopathic remedy is to take *Baryta muriatica 6c* three times a day for three weeks and *Proteus 30c* during attacks.

Herbalists recommend an infusion made from hawthorn berries to improve the circulatory system. Pour one cup of boiling water over 1 tablespoon of berries; steep for 20 minutes. Drink two to three times a day.

VARICOSE VEINS

Blood returning from the feet and legs to the heart has a long, hard climb against the pull of gravity. To help it on its way and prevent excess pressure on the walls of the vessels at the bottom of the system, the veins are divided into short sections by one-way valves, which allow the blood to move only upward. If the valves in the deep veins of the legs begin to fail, blood is forced back into the surface veins, which swell, twist, and stretch under the pressure, causing the blue/red swellings known as varicose veins. (Varicose veins that occur in or around the anal area are known as hemorrhoids.)

Varicose veins are more common in women than men. Pregnancy, being overweight, and work that involves standing for extended periods of time all tend to increase the risk of developing the condition.

Symptoms

Some people with varicose veins experience aching, swollen, and tired legs, and, in severe cases, develop skin rashes and ulcers. But for many there is no discomfort or pain. The principal concern is the appearance of the legs because the affected veins become blue, twisted, and prominent.

Treatment

In mild cases of varicose veins, using elastic support stockings and, if possible, standing still for less time and doing more walking is enough to relieve symptoms. Lying down and raising the legs helps relieve swelling.

A procedure known as sclerotherapy can also be performed, in which a blood clot is artificially created in the vein by injection of a chemical solution. The clot blocks the varicose vein, causing blood to be diverted through unaffected veins.

In severe cases surgery is the only long-term answer. This is done in one of two ways. A long wire is threaded through the vein from the groin to the ankle and the vein is tied to it and then pulled out, a procedure called stripping. Alternatively, the small veins connecting the affected superficial veins to the deep veins can be cut and tied off.

Natural therapies

Naturopaths recommend vitamin E and C supplements for their antioxidant properties. Extracts of horse chestnut are recommended by herbalists; this herb has been shown to reduce edema as effectively as support stockings and improve the tone of veins by helping the walls to better contract. And certain herbal remedies can relieve discomfort and pain. For example, you can make a soothing poultice from marigold flowers. Gotu kola and ginkgo biloba tablets will help improve circulation; these are available in pharmacies and health food stores.

Homeopathic remedies, *Pulsatilla, Carbo veg,* and *Lycopodium,* may also improve circulation. Consult a homeopath.

Certain yoga (see page 104) exercises help improve circulation as well. You can adopt the following posture to relieve pressure on your legs: Lie at a right angle to a wall and place your feet up against it with your hips as close to the wall as possible. Stay in this position for at least three minutes every day.

Hydrotherapy, too, is useful for stimulating circulation. Fill one basin with hot water and another with cold water and ice cubes. Soak a towel in each basin and wring it out. Place the hot towel on the vein for a minute, then the cold one for 30 seconds. Repeat three times, ending with the cold towel.

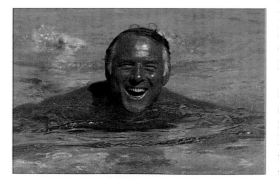

SWIMMING
Swimming is the ideal exercise for someone whose varicose veins make walking painful. It also improves general circulation and strengthens the heart.

CHAPTER 7

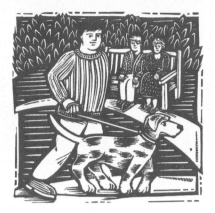

THE ROAD TO RECOVERY

The pain and shock of a heart attack or heart surgery might spur you to change your life for the better. Coming close to death often provides the motivation to adopt a healthier lifestyle. Rehabilitation, under the guidance of health professionals, involves adopting a healthier diet, following a supervised exercise program, and learning stress and anger management techniques.

SPEEDING YOUR RECOVERY

Many patients claim that they feel better after recovering from a heart attack or heart surgery than they have for many years, possibly because of a new lifestyle and readjustment of priorities.

RISKY BUSINESS

After a heart attack, you can do almost everything you could do before. But there are a few activities you should avoid.

▶ *Do not run for buses. Regular exercise is good for you, but sudden exertion is not.*

▶ *Avoid heavy digging in the garden.*

▶ *Rest for half an hour after eating or having a hot bath, and avoid doing the two activities within two hours of each other. Take showers instead of baths whenever possible.*

▶ *Do not carry heavy objects, such as luggage, even for short distances.*

▶ *Do not push yourself beyond your limits; know when to stop.*

Full recovery from a heart attack or bypass surgery usually takes two to three months. As you resume normal life during this time, your emotions and physical capabilities will go through several changes. Once you are out of the hospital, and gradually recuperating at home, you may decide to institute changes in lifestyle that will ensure future health.

The speed and extent of recovery from a heart attack will depend on the amount of physical damage that has occurred. Heart muscle that has died does not regrow, so any damage is permanent.

Location of the damage is also an important factor. A small amount of dead muscle in a vital position, for instance at the base of a heart valve or in an area vital to the heart's internal electrical system, can cause greater disability than a larger amount of dead muscle in a less important position. If part of your heart has been impaired, it is essential to prevent further damage from

RELAX AND REST
If you have trouble sleeping, ask your partner to give you a shoulder rub. It is an effective way to relieve tension and anxiety.

occurring and to minimize the strain on your heart. Similarly, if you have had bypass surgery, you will have to take actions to recover your health and prevent further harm to your arteries.

THE NEED FOR SLEEP

Sleep is a vital part of the process of healing. At first you may find yourself sleeping 10 to 12 hours each night, as well as taking a nap of 2 hours or more every afternoon. This is not unusual; often people need more sleep for about a year after a heart attack. But since you will almost certainly feel worried and anxious, sleep may not come easily or be completely restful.

If you have trouble getting to sleep, try taking a warm (not hot) bath before bedtime, drinking an herbal tea with a sedative effect, such as chamomile or valerian, or doing relaxation exercises (see page 82). Many people find that they sleep better after a massage. Ask your partner to massage your shoulders or rub your back with some lavender-scented oil to help you drop off.

ACTIVITY IS IMPORTANT

Paradoxically, while you need more rest, your body also needs to remain active. Many people are surprised by how soon the hospital staff encourages them to get out of bed. Prolonged bed rest actually weakens muscles. After only three weeks in bed, even a healthy person loses one-third of his or her strength, and regaining that strength will take a few weeks. Lung infections are also common in people confined to bed for long periods. Cardiologists therefore recommend getting up and sitting in a chair or even walking with the aid of a nurse a day or two after a heart attack. A week later you may be climbing stairs or taking a shower alone, depending on the severity of your heart attack and the advice of your doctor.

But all activity, and exercise in particular, must begin gradually. After a heart attack the damaged heart muscle must form a scar, which takes about six weeks. During that time you must not exert yourself any more than your doctor allows and should do everything that he or she recommends.

You will have to walk this fine line between doing too much and not doing enough during the entire period of your recovery. Your best guides are the advice of your physician or cardiac rehabilitation manager and what your own body is telling you. Listen to your body. If you feel tired, stop what you are doing and rest.

UNDERSTANDING YOUR EMOTIONS

Heart trouble often leads to a troubled heart. You may feel that a part of you died in the heart attack. A heart attack causes psychological damage to a degree not seen with many other forms of illness. The heart is more than a mere biological pump. It has an especially important position in people's perceptions of themselves, a significance reflected in all human language and culture, particularly as the center of love.

A number of patients find themselves asking, "Why me?" Others lash out in anger and frustration at their partners and families. Although this anger is very common, it is also very damaging, because anger and stress cause both blood pressure and cholesterol levels to rise. It is important to learn to control anger (see page 152).

Many people feel let down by their bodies. Depression is a common reaction, as well as insomnia and a general lethargy and lack of interest in life. If these symptoms are severe or persist for more than a week or two after you get out of the hospital, you should talk to your doctor about getting counseling. Also, you should start learning stress management techniques (see page 150).

Overcoming depression

To overcome the mild depression that is most common after a heart attack or heart surgery, you have to become optimistic about your recovery, recognizing that most people who survive a heart attack go on to lead normal lives. People with optimistic attitudes are the ones who take control of their lives and begin the steps that will lead them back to health.

The first step in the healing process is to acknowledge that you have heart disease. (Surprisingly, many people refuse to face this fact.) Next, you must recognize that although you will never be cured of heart disease, you can learn to control it through diet, exercise, and stress management.

CHANGE YOUR DIET

The dietary advice for heart patients is the same as it is for everyone else: eat more fruits, vegetables, and whole grains and fewer fatty foods like meat, oil, butter, and cheese. Because most heart disease is caused by clogged arteries, you have an added incentive to change bad eating habits—to prevent another heart attack. If you are overweight, you will also need to lose weight. A low-fat diet will help you not only to do this but also to maintain a lower weight. (See Chapter 3 for more information on eating for a healthy heart.)

Caffeine and alcohol

Both alcohol and caffeine should be consumed only in moderation. Taken in excess, alcohol can raise your blood pressure and caffeine can cause palpitations.

continued on page 136

Diet for depression

There is some evidence that the amino acid tryptophan relieves depression because it is used by the body to make serotonin, a chemical that is essential for various processes in the brain that involve moods.

Tryptophan is found in milk, fish, peanut butter, nuts, and cooked dried beans and peas. Eating any of these foods together with cereal foods like bread, pasta, and rice facilitates the uptake of tryptophan in the brain.

SELF-HELP FOR DEPRESSION

Survivors of heart attacks often feel depressed and at a loss as to how to piece their lives back together. Acupressure and aromatherapy can be helpful in overcoming depression.

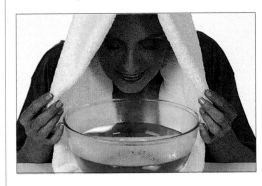

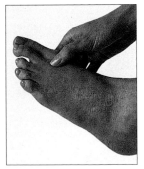

AROMATHERAPY
Put three drops of clary sage or jasmine essential oil into a basin of steaming water. Cover your head with a towel and inhale. Or put 6 drops of the oil onto a handkerchief and inhale.

ACUPRESSURE
Point Liv 3: two finger widths toward the ankle from the junction of the big and second toes.

A Recovering Cardiac Case

Having a coronary artery bypass is often a turning point in a person's life and the first step on a path to recovery. With modern knowledge about the factors that cause coronary heart disease and ever more advanced surgical techniques, thousands of patients have become living testimonials to the fact that heart disease can have a happy ending.

Tom is a 51-year-old freelance computer consultant who set up his own business six years ago after being laid off from a large multinational company. His wife, Alison, is an elementary school teacher, and they have two children—Sarah, who has just finished college and is looking for a job in marketing, and Nick, who is still in college studying for his electrical engineering degree.

Following Tom's layoff, the family income dropped dramatically. It became necessary to remortgage their house, and the children's university expenses have severely taxed their income, causing Tom and Alison many sleepless nights.

Tom was diagnosed with angina at age 43, and he was so frightened that he gave up smoking and went on a weight-loss and exercise program. Although he lost 4.5 kg (10 lb) fairly quickly, Tom has found it difficult to keep the weight off. A couple of weeks after the diagnosis, he also had balloon angioplasty (see page 111) to clear a severely blocked coronary artery. He has been on anti-angina medication ever since, but the angina attacks have continued, which has worried them.

Tom and Alison are concerned about his health because his father died of a heart attack at the age of 67. Their relationship has become strained because they see no solution to their financial problems. Tom's freelance earnings are not enough to keep them out of trouble.

Tom had a coronary angiogram a few weeks ago that showed extensive narrowing in three of his coronary arteries. On the cardiac surgeon's recommendation, he had coronary artery bypass surgery (see page 112), and stayed in the hospital for a week after the operation.

FAMILY
Marital relations can suffer when one member's health difficulties become exacerbated by financial considerations. Professional guidance may be needed to work through the problems.

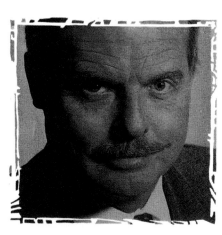

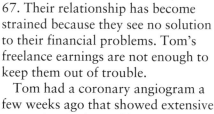

EXERCISE
A patient who has had heart surgery must begin exercise as soon as possible to improve cardiovascular efficiency.

DIET
Staying on a low-fat, high-fiber diet is essential for preventing fatty deposits in any more arteries.

WORK
Self-employment can be particularly stressful if financial security is at stake, and it may be difficult to take time off after an operation.

HEALTH
To avoid further heart problems, it is necessary to make appropriate lifestyle changes that include a healthier diet, a reduction in alcohol, regular exercise, and stress management.

WHAT SHOULD TOM DO?

Tom has now been discharged from the hospital and must follow the doctor's instructions carefully. He has been told to rest often at first but to resume gentle activity as soon as he is able. However, he should not go out on cold or windy days.

Tom is also not allowed to drive for at least four weeks, and if he travels as a passenger, he should pad the seat belt, but definitely wear it! He should not lift anything heavy and must avoid all strenuous activity.

Adhering carefully to his rehabilitation program—which has been devised by a team of cardiologists, nurses, physiotherapists, occupational therapists, a psychologist, a pharmacist, a dietitian, and his own primary care physician—is essential. To help him in this effort he has been given a daily activity sheet. The recommended regimen includes a low-fat diet prescribed by the dietitian and regular practice of relaxation exercises.

He is encouraged to discuss all worries with the team psychologist, not just concerns about his health but also those that relate to family, financial matters, and his business. He and Alison must also seek solutions to their financial problems in order to reduce the stresses on them both. They should discuss the entire situation with their children and ask them to help out.

Action Plan

DIET
Eat low-fat meals and plenty of fresh fruits and vegetables. Avoid sugary foods. Eat small amounts several times a day rather than large meals. Have mimimal alcohol. Follow all instructions given by the dietitian.

EXERCISE
Do leg and breathing exercises at home as instructed. Walk daily but don't overdo it. Dress comfortably and be careful not to become cold. Visit the physiotherapist weekly.

FAMILY
Talk to Alison about any concerns, including feelings of depression. Ask the children to assist with household tasks to minimize stress on Alison. Go to counseling with Alison to discuss worries and anxiety. Ask for advice about resuming sexual relations.

HEALTH
Follow diet and exercise programs carefully and monitor progress. Do relaxation exercises daily to relieve stress.

WORK
Initially, take on only small jobs. Don't agree to deadlines that will prove difficult to meet and cause extra stress. Get assistance if necessary. Talk to the bank about possibly refinancing the mortgage again. Ask Nick to look for a part-time job at school and a full-time job during the summer.

HOW THINGS TURNED OUT FOR TOM

Tom experienced chest discomfort and some pain for several weeks after the operation. His doctor prescribed painkillers. On the day after he arrived home from the hospital, Tom was able to sit in a chair, and the following day he moved around the house a little. By the second week he started walking daily, gradually increasing his distance over the next few weeks. He rested every afternoon and did not have too many visitors.

He followed a low-fat diet that included more fruits and vegetables than before. Tom discussed his feelings of depression with the team psychologist and practiced relaxation exercises at home. The physiotherapist assisted Tom with breathing exercises to prevent mucus buildup in his lungs and leg exercises to improve his circulation. Alison attended parts of the rehabilitation course with him, so she could give him support. After a

few weeks he began to return to normal daily activities. His angina disappeared, and his improved health helped restore their relationship. They resumed sexual relations after six weeks.

After two months Tom began to take small freelance assignments, making sure he did not agree to anything with very tight deadlines. Alison continued to work and Sarah and Nick found jobs, which eased the financial strain a little.

Driving a car

Many people worry about driving safely following a heart attack. Doctors recommend that patients who have been hospitalized not drive for at least four weeks after being discharged, depending on the severity of the problem and side effects of any medications. This is because their condition may not be stable enough for them to drive safely, medications may affect their alertness, and driving itself may cause too much stress.

You should limit caffeinated drinks (tea, coffee, and cola) to two per day. If you are a heavy tea or coffee drinker, you could try changing gradually to decaffeinated beverages. Herbal teas are also healthful, and some of them—chamomile and valerian, for instance—are particularly relaxing.

Although some studies have shown that alcohol, especially red wine, may have a protective effect on the heart (see page 64), more than two drinks a day is harmful (see page 119). Too much alcohol will also hinder your weight-loss program. If you are on medication for your heart or blood pressure, it may be necessary to avoid alcohol altogether. Consult with your doctor

BUILDING UP FITNESS

Generally, you will be advised to begin with gentle walking and to avoid walking either up or down hill. You are allowed to exercise out of doors but should avoid doing so in extreme weather conditions. Along with a low-fat diet, regular exercise is probably the most important thing you can do to keep your arteries clear.

Many hospitals now run cardiac rehabilitation programs. If your hospital does not have one, ask if there is one in your area that you can join. These programs provide a structured setting in which you can build up your physical strength, find out how to make the necessary changes in your diet, and learn to control stress. They are beneficial for people of all ages.

Cardiac rehabilitation programs are usually organized in four phases. In Phase I you are in the hospital recovering from a cardiac event. In Phase II you recover at home. This can take between two and six weeks. During Phase III, you attend a rehabilitation center for regular exercise and education sessions until your optimal physical condition is achieved. This often takes from 6 to 12 weeks. When you enter Phase IV, you are no longer a patient but are back in the community attending a support group or fitness club, although you may still be in touch with your cardiac rehabilitation manager (see page 138).

Whether you join a cardiac rehabilitation group or not, you should exercise regularly, gradually increasing the time and intensity. You can discuss the appropriate amount and type of exercise with your doctor or a physiotherapist. You may feel breathless when you begin exercising, possibly because you were out of shape before your heart attack or bypass surgery, or because you still have some lingering heart problems. It is important to tell your doctor about any episodes of breathlessness.

One of the best forms of exercise for heart patients is simply taking a 20-minute walk

CARDIAC REHABILITATION EXERCISES

Phase I of a cardiac rehabilitation program takes place when you are still in the hospital following a heart attack or heart surgery. During this time, care must be taken to avoid strain or exertion, and the doctor's instructions must be followed. The following exercises are advised in Phase I, when it is important to start moving a little, but you should be very careful not to overexert yourself. These exercises are usually followed by walking increasing distances around the hospital building and then up and down stairs.

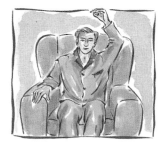

ARM LIFTS
Sitting in a chair, lift your arms up one at a time. If you feel up to it, you should do these arm lifts while standing.

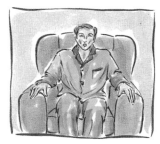

DEEP BREATHING
Take in deep, relaxed breaths, making sure that your abdomen rises and falls with each one.

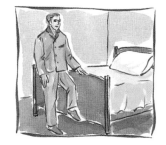

KNEE BENDS
Do alternate knee bends while holding onto the bed. Walk around the bed if you are up to it.

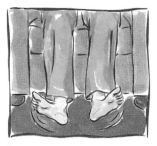

ANKLE STRETCH
When sitting down, move your ankles side to side and in circles to stimulate circulation in the legs.

HEALING YOUR HEART WITH VISUALIZATION

You can use your mind and imagination to help your heart heal. Creative visualization is often used by cancer patients to imagine their bodies fighting off the cancer cells. Heart patients can use the same technique. Simply set aside some time when you can sit quietly without being disturbed. Close your eyes and relax, then picture your heart and try to visualize its problem. Perhaps is has blockage in the arteries or scars from your surgery. Think about the kind of healing your heart needs. Are the arteries full of plaque that needs to be washed away? You might imagine an army of tiny cleaners scrubbing away the debris. Spend some time thinking about the image in detail. After a few minutes, open your eyes and take a few deep breaths. Doing this healing exercise for 10 minutes every day should help you feel more in control of your recovery.

every day. But make sure you warm up and stretch adequately before you do any exercise (see Chapter 4), including walking. It is essential to go for regular check-ups with your doctor to assess whether your physical fitness is improving satisfactorily.

It is also a good idea to record your progress by keeping an exercise journal, writing down what you did every day and how you felt. Then, on days when you become discouraged, you can look back and see how far you have come.

RESUMING SEXUAL RELATIONS

Many people want to know when they can begin sexual activity again, but are too shy to ask their doctors. And many doctors, particularly when talking to older people, neglect to give advice on this issue.

Cause for anxiety

Following a heart attack or heart surgery, most people resume their sex lives as before. For some patients, however, their medications or anxiety about triggering a heart attack can make sex difficult. Talking to your doctor can help. He or she can determine whether or not your medication could

be causing problems (such as failure to become aroused). Your doctor will also be able to reassure you that very few people die during lovemaking. This is because making love is in most cases not a particularly strenuous form of physical exertion.

Proceed with caution

When resuming sexual relations after a heart attack or surgery, proceed slowly and gently. Do not make love after eating a heavy meal or having an alcoholic drink; both will make your heart beat faster, and any exertion will put it under more strain. Instead, try making love in the morning when you are well rested or in the afternoon after a nap. Begin by gently touching and caressing one another. If you want to proceed to intercourse, find a position that feels comfortable—the missionary, or man on top position, can put too much stress on the man's upper body and on the woman's chest. Instead, try sex side by side, from the rear, or with the woman on top. Many experts recommend simply touching, kissing, and hugging. This provides physical closeness without the anxiety that heart patients sometimes feel during sex.

If you find, despite these recommendations, that your sex life does not return to normal or that you continue to have problems with arousal, you may need a change in your existing medication. A sex therapist may be able to help if problems persist.

Contact your doctor if you experience any of the following warning signs: breathlessness or rapid heartbeat for more than 15 minutes after sex; feeling exceptionally tired immediately after sex or on the following day; chest pain or discomfort during sex; heartbeat irregularities during or after sex; and insomnia during the night after sex.

Smokers must quit
Smokers have only half as much chance of surviving short-term and long-term after a heart attack as nonsmokers. Yet half of all smokers who have had heart attacks continue to smoke. Of those who quit after bypass surgery, between 40 and 75 percent start smoking again.

Quitting smoking is always difficult, but in the aftermath of a heart attack it can be doubly so. You are anxious, irritable, and depressed and may feel that you need cigarettes more than ever. Also, you are struggling with making changes in so many areas of your life that quitting smoking may seem impossible. But it is vital to your survival. See page 36 for helpful ideas on how to quit smoking.

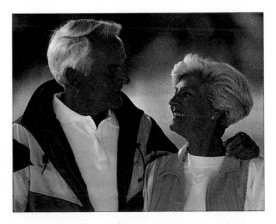

*BEING AFFECTIONATE
A heart attack or surgery takes a lot out of you. Instead of rushing into sex, you can try other ways of being intimate until you feel ready for it.*

Rehabilitation Manager

The aim of cardiac rehabilitation is to restore cardiac patients to reasonable physical health and quality of life and to promote changes in lifestyle to reduce the risks of further heart problems. The cardiac rehabilitation manager supervises this approach.

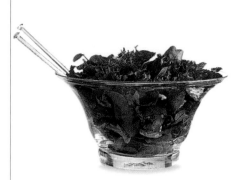

A NEW DIET
Changing your eating habits is essential for recovering from a heart attack. A cardiac rehabilitation manager, together with a dietitian or nutritionist, can help you learn the best way to cut down on fat and eat the right nutritious food.

CARDIAC REHABILITATION
Exercise (see page 136) is a vital part of all rehabilitation phases but should always be supervised. During phase I you are recovering in the hospital. In Phase II you are at home. Phase III involves regular visits to a rehabilitation center until you are fit, and in Phase IV you are no longer a patient but may be attending a support group.

A rehabilitation program has four phases, beginning with the time spent in the hospital and ending with a return to normal life. The initial focus is on physical exercises to restore health and develop the ability of the damaged heart to function as effectively as possible. But other risk factors, such as smoking, a high-fat diet, heavy drinking, and excessive stress, must be addressed as well. Also, psychological and sexual problems may have to be dealt with.

What does a cardiac rehabilitation manager do?
The manager assesses each patient's needs and, together with the patient's doctor, devises a suitable program for him or her from the courses and specialists available. The manager monitors progress and makes adjustments and referrals as required.

Who is involved in rehabilitation?
A core team is made up of nurses and physiotherapists or occupational therapists, with supervision from consultant cardiologists and other physicians. The team may also include a dietitian, a stress management counselor, a pharmacist, a psychologist, and an exercise specialist.

A rehabilitation manager may refer a patient to a sex therapist, social worker, vocational counselor, or other specialist as well.

What training does a manager have?
A rehabilitation manager is often a cardiac nurse or physiotherapist who is familiar with all the disciplines involved in a cardiac program and is fully trained in advanced cardiopulmonary resuscitation.

Who benefits from rehabilitation?
Research shows that most people who have suffered a cardiac event will benefit from rehabilitation. The term "cardiac event" covers heart attacks, heart failure, and all heart surgery, including transplants. Patients suffering from less severe heart problems can also benefit. Approximately three-quarters of the patients who have been through a cardiac rehabilitation program stay well and active for five or more years after their cardiac event, as opposed to only half of those who have not been in a program.

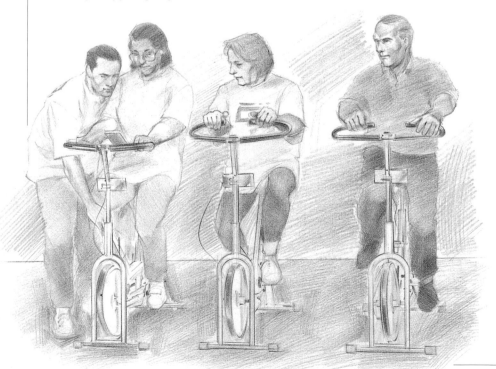

How does the exercise component work?

A rehabilitation doctor will give you exercise tests at each phase to assess how well your heart is functioning and to evaluate the effects of your training. Until the heart muscle has healed, a patient should not exercise strenuously. Therefore, during Phase II, a regimen of incremental brisk walking (where the distance covered is gradually increased) is usually the only exercise advised.

Phase III usually consists of several group exercise sessions per week under medical supervision, with equivalent sessions at home on the other days of the week. The sequence includes aerobic exercises to get the cardiovascular system working as well as possible, strength exercises to develop the major muscle groups so that you can live a normal life, and flexibility exercises to help prevent other problems from developing, such as in the back and joints.

Ex-cardiac patients are encouraged in Phase IV to join support groups, which meet regularly to take part in exercise classes and discussion sessions. A rehabilitation manager may keep in touch through the group and is available for further advice or referral if required.

What does education include?

During Phase I, a rehabilitation manager will visit you to explain the rehabilitation process, talk about your work and home situation, and find out about particular problems you may have. You may be given booklets or attend seminars in the hospital that explain cardiac anatomy and disease and give advice about medication. Seminars allow you to ask questions and discuss fears and problems. Former cardiac patients may also take part to offer the benefit of their experience.

During Phase III, various education sessions are usually given on cardiac risk factors, especially diet, stress, and smoking. These are often structured discussion groups lead by an appropriate specialist.

Can my family be involved?

It is vital for close family or friends to be involved in your rehabilitation and to have a full understanding of the phases, to relieve their own anxiety about your illness, as well as to aid your recovery. They can help you to eat and exercise sensibly, support you in giving up smoking, and bolster you during a low point. If you are having job, emotional, or sexual problems, your partner or caregiver may be asked to join you in some counseling or therapy sessions.

During Phase III, partners or other close family members are encouraged to attend the education sessions. When you graduate to Phase IV, it is helpful for your partner to join the support groups, too, and to share exercise activities. Apart from the exercises being fun to do together, they may also benefit your partner's health and well-being and help you both to relieve stress.

Is stress management important?

Learning about stress management is a vital part of cardiac rehabilitation. Stress management enables you to relieve tension before it causes further cardiac damage by teaching you relaxation and creative activities.

Does cardiac rehabilitation help with psychological problems?

Talking to your rehabilitation manager or team, and to former patients and other patients in your program, can help immensely. Simply finding out that other people have the same problems can be reassuring. For example, it is very common to feel far more emotional than usual during phases I and II. If you are suffering from depression or excessive anger, your manager can refer you to a psychologist. The regular weekly sessions are individual and confidential.

What about sexual problems?

Difficulties with resuming sexual activities are common, especially after cardiac surgery (see page 137). The rehabilitation manager may refer you to a sex therapist, who will then determine the nature of your sexual problem and help you solve it.

What about work problems?

The rehabilitation team can teach you exercises specifically designed to get you back to work. The manager can inform your employer when you are ready to return to work. If you have lost your job because of your illness, the rehabilitation manager may be able to help get you reinstated.

If your condition prevents you from continuing in your previous work, the manager can refer you for vocational counseling, so that you can explore other options and also investigate any opportunities for further training.

If you support dependent family members, you may also be referred to a social worker, who can advise you on benefits you are entitled to and arrange for extra help in the home.

WHAT YOU CAN DO AT HOME

Here are some pointers to help you during the first couple of weeks after coming out of the hospital.

▶ *Keep a daily diary of your physical and mental progress.*

▶ *Listen to your body and do not push yourself if you are having a low day.*

▶ *Use a relaxation tape and/or soothing music as part of your daily routine.*

RELAXATION
When you are feeling stressed or negative, listen to some soothing music.

CONTROLLING BLOOD PRESSURE

Following a diagnosis of heart disease or after any kind of heart surgery, it is essential to reduce high blood pressure with lifestyle changes and, if necessary, medication.

CALM YOUR BLOOD PRESSURE DOWN

Try the following measures to help you lower your blood pressure in nonmedical ways.

▶ *Smile more.*

▶ *Laugh a lot.*

▶ *Chat with a friend.*

▶ *Pet an animal.*

▶ *Buy yourself a present.*

▶ *Read a book or magazine.*

▶ *Have a scented bath.*

▶ *Think positive thoughts.*

▶ *Chase negative thoughts away.*

PET THERAPY
Research has shown that interacting with a pet lowers blood pressure and is relaxing and comforting as well.

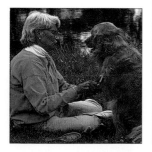

High blood pressure greatly increases the risk of developing heart disease because it increases formation of atheromas. As arteries become narrower from plaques (see page 108), high blood pressure may cause the plaques to break. The damaged wall will then bleed and a clot will form. The clot could become large enough to obstruct the artery completely.

High blood pressure can also increase the severity of aneurysms (see page 129) and cause strokes (see page 127).

Following a heart attack, heart surgery, or a diagnosis of a heart or circulatory disorder, if your blood pressure is dangerously high or you are at a very high risk of having another heart attack, your doctor may prescribe medication. Although medications offer lifesaving benefits, these drugs can also have unpleasant side effects, such as impotence, fatigue, and depression. Some doctors estimate that as many as 90 percent of their patients do not bother to take their medication, perhaps because they are discouraged by the side effects.

MAKING CHANGES

In addition to prescribing drug therapy, doctors encourage their patients to make adjustments in their way of life—changing what they eat, the amount they exercise, and the way they deal with stress.

As with all heart-related problems, a low-fat diet and moderate aerobic exercise are recommended to reduce blood pressure. Quitting smoking is also advised (see page 34). If you are overweight it is important to lose pounds. Stress management is also essential. All these changes, followed rigorously, can lower blood pressure and enable a patient to reduce or forgo medication.

THE STRESS CONNECTION

Blood pressure is linked closely to the emotions, as evidenced by a phenomenon known as "white-coat hypertension," which results in higher than usual blood pressure readings at the doctor's office. If just a simple visit to the doctor can raise your blood pressure, imagine how much more it is raised by all the hassles of daily life: family disputes, traffic jams, and pressure at work. Reducing anxiety by avoiding stressful situations whenever possible and changing how you react to unavoidable stress can be helpful in keeping blood pressure from rising.

Stress reduction

Learning how to relax can help lower your blood pressure by a few points. You can use a progressive relaxation method (see page 82) or take up yoga or meditation (see page 104). These methods not only lower blood pressure while you are using them, but they also foster lower blood pressure throughout the day and carry lasting benefits.

Massage can be a great aid to relaxation. When used in combination with aromatherapy (see page 100), it can be particularly beneficial in lowering blood pressure. A trained aromatherapist will use certain essential oils that enhance the effects.

Biofeedback has shown dramatic results in lowering blood pressure. A study done at St. Luke's Hospital in New York in 1989 examined the effect of biofeedback on 30 patients who had had hypertension for at least two years. After learning biofeedback techniques, their blood pressure fell to within the normal range.

The results of another study, reported in the *British Medical Journal* in 1981, showed that a group of 200 workers with high blood pressure were able to reduce it dramatically by using relaxation and biofeedback alone. Eight months later they were still benefiting from the training.

THE DIET CONNECTION
There are foods you will be told to steer clear of to lower your blood pressure, such as those high in saturated fat. Most doctors also recommend lowering intake of sodium, by not adding salt to food at the table and avoiding processed foods that are high in salt and other sodium compounds (see page 51). In addition, you may be advised to eat certain foods that are known to help keep blood pressure normal.

Mineral magic
Three minerals besides sodium are involved in the regulation of blood pressure—potassium, magnesium, and calcium. Deficiencies of any of these may cause hypertension. Such deficiencies can occur, in part, from taking diuretic medications for lowering blood presssure because diuretics cause minerals to be excreted in the urine.

The best way to obtain these minerals is through your diet. Most plant foods contain at least some potassium, but bananas, citrus fruits, tomatoes, potatoes, legumes, green vegetables, and whole grains are especially rich sources. Magnesium is plentiful in many foods, including leafy greens, legumes, seeds, nuts, and whole grains. Calcium is found in dairy products, tofu, leafy green vegetables, some fruits, nuts, and seeds, and the bones of canned fish. In general, the calcium in milk and soft fish bones is more easily absorbed than that in plants. (Low-fat or nonfat dairy products should be used to minimize intake of saturated fats.)

Mineral supplements may be of additional benefit in some cases. In one study, women who received 800 mg of calcium supplements per day had a 23 percent decrease in their blood pressure. Some studies involving supplementation of potassium and magnesium have also showed reductions in blood pressure. However, mineral supplements can be dangerous, especially for people with severe kidney or heart problems. A doctor's supervision is essential.

Walking your blood pressure down
Exercise is one of the most effective ways of reducing blood pressure without medication. A study reported in *Harvard Health Letter* in February 1995 revealed that moderate walking (20 to 30 minutes three times per week) lowers blood pressure. Older people and anyone with a medical condition should consult a doctor before starting a walking program.

LOWERING BLOOD PRESSURE WITH BIOFEEDBACK TRAINING

Biofeedback training is a way of gaining a measure of control over bodily functions that are usually automatic, or involuntary, such as blood pressure, skin temperature, heartbeat, even brain-wave patterns.

With electronic sensors a biofeedback machine measures muscle activity, brain waves, or galvanic skin response (GSR—the activity of sweat glands and skin temperature), while a monitor indicates changes in these involuntary bodily functions by a sound, flashing light, or picture on a screen. During biofeedback training, patients learn how to alter the electronic signals and, in the process, change an involuntary response that is detrimental to their health or well-being, thus becoming active participants in their treatment.

The training may be done by a physician, psychologist, physical therapist, or a laboratory technician, often in a rehabilitation center.

Biofeedback is commonly used to control chronic pain, rehabilitate muscles damaged by stroke, and treat stress-related conditions like migraine headaches and high blood pressure. It has also been used in a heart-attack prevention program to modify persistent feelings of anger and hostility, which are thought to increase the risk of heart attack.

Biofeedback training may include deep breathing, progressive muscular relaxation, autohypnotic suggestion, creative visualization, and meditation or a combination of these techniques. Seeing the image on the screen or hearing the signal, a patient will employ these methods to relax muscles. Eventually, a patient is able to achieve the desired results without the presence of the machine

In many cases biofeedback can reduce or eliminate the need for medications. It can also foster a feeling of increased well-being.

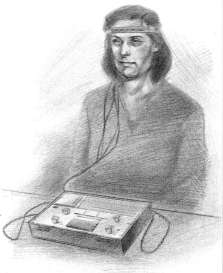

MONITORING YOURSELF
Using biofeedback, you can monitor your muscle tension, fluctuations in skin temperature, and changes in blood pressure. Through relaxation exercises you can then influence these physiological factors.

CHANGING YOUR EATING HABITS

Dietary changes are essential for anyone who has a heart or circulatory problem. The right diet can not only prevent further damage to arteries but may also reverse some existing damage.

Energy requirements
To lose weight you must burn more calories than you eat. The chart below, right, provides a guide to the calories required for different levels of activity. Note that these are estimates; if you are ill, pregnant, or breast-feeding, your doctor will probably make different recommendations.

The dietary advice for treating heart disease is very similar to that for preventing heart problems (see chapter 3). Changing your diet can help prevent further damage to your arteries.

Many people worry that they don't have the willpower to change their eating habits, but once they have tried a healthier diet and realize how much better they feel, willpower is usually not a problem. Newly established changes can be reinforced, nonetheless, by keeping only healthful foods in the house to avoid temptation.

WEIGHT CONTROL

It is important for anyone with heart problems to be in the normal weight range for their height (see page 97). Being overweight is linked to increased blood pressure, raised blood cholesterol levels, and adult-onset diabetes. All of these conditions can lead to heart disease and are much easier to control if some excess weight is lost.

Your doctor may be able to advise you on where to get help with losing weight. Some dietitians run weight-loss programs for a fixed period of time, which may be enough

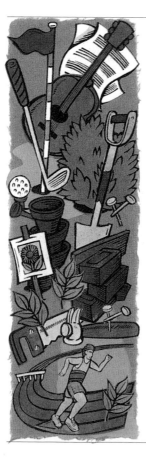

DAILY ENERGY REQUIREMENTS

You can calculate your daily calorie requirements with this chart. First figure out which activity category you fit into, then multiply your weight by the figure given. The figures represent calories per kilogram (kg) of body weight. (If your scale weighs in pounds, divide by 2.2 to calculate kg.)

ACTIVITY	MEN (calories per kg body weight)	WOMEN (calories per kg body weight)
VERY LIGHT		
Office work, cooking, sewing, playing musical instruments	31	30
LIGHT		
Strolling, cleaning, shopping, golf	38	35
MODERATE		
Fast walking, gardening, bicycling, skiing, tennis, dancing	41	37
HEAVY		
Manual labor, rock climbing, team sports	50	44
EXTRA HEAVY		
Athletic training	58	51

EATING AWAY FROM HOME

Having a heart problem can be a special challenge when away from home. No matter what situation you find yourself in, you don't have an excuse to abandon your healthy diet.

Avoid, if possible, going to fast-food restaurants that serve mainly high-fat hamburgers, hotdogs, and french fries. Milk shakes and creamy desserts are also absolutely loaded with fat. If there is no alternative, choose a salad and use a dressing sparingly.

In restaurants order steamed, stir-fried, grilled, or baked dishes instead of fried ones. And avoid creamy soups and sauces. Get into the habit of asking the waiter questions. You can also ask for vegetarian or low-fat alternatives.

If you are traveling by air, request a vegetarian, fat-free, diabetic, or low-salt meal. Make sure you order it when you book your ticket.

When you are invited to the home of friends, always tell them about your special diet needs and offer to bring something with you. This saves you from refusing their food or indulging and feeling guilty.

to get you started. Otherwise, think about joining a self-help group for weight control, but make sure the people who run the program are aware of your medical history.

Be careful about any weight-loss program that promises amazing results or sells liquid meals or nutritional supplements as part of the regimen; most of these plans work only in the short-term or not at all, and some supplements may not be suitable for you to take along with your heart medication.

An effective weight-reducing program combines diet changes with an increase in exercise. The amount and intensity of exercise suitable for heart patients varies according to their physical condition. Cardiac rehabilitation programs for patients who have had a heart attack or surgery usually include a daily walk to start—with a gradual increase in the time and pace. A routine that increases muscle mass as well as aerobic fitness will help raise the rate at which you burn calories. You can check what is right for you with your doctor.

LOWERING CHOLESTEROL

Anyone with a heart or circulatory problem may have to reduce his or her cholesterol levels because high cholesterol is a major factor in the formation of arterial plaques that lead to heart disease. It also contributes to the development of blood clots (see page 125), as well as such arterial diseases as intermittent claudication (see page 129).

Most people can reduce their cholesterol through dietary measures. These include reducing both total and saturated fat (the best effects, so far, have been achieved with diets that contain only 10 percent total fat), limiting intake of cholesterol to 300 milligrams a day (about the amount in 1½ egg yolks), and including more soluble fiber and oily fish in the diet. It is believed that fiber may help lower cholesterol by interfering with the intestinal absorption of bile acids, which forces the liver to use circulating cholesterol to make more bile.

A cholesterol-lowering diet works best when combined with an exercise program. Regular exercise helps increase blood levels of "good" HDL cholesterol and lower the levels of "bad" LDL cholesterol (see page 38). As always, check with your doctor about the level and amount of activity.

When diet and exercise fail to lower cholesterol to acceptable levels, cholesterol-lowering medication may be necessary, particularly for people who have a family history of high cholesterol (see page 32).

LOWERING TRIGLYCERIDES

Triglycerides are another type of dietary and blood lipid (fat) that, like cholesterol, play an important role in many bodily functions. They carry the fat-soluble vitamins A, D, E, and K and help synthesize certain hormones. However, some evidence points to a high triglyceride level—above 200 milligrams—as a factor in heart disease, especially when the level of HDL lipoproteins is correspondingly low.

An accurate triglyceride reading can be obtained only after a fast of at least 12 hours. If your blood test shows elevated triglycerides, you will need to reduce them. To lower triglycerides, lose weight and limit intake of alcohol and foods that are high in saturated fat and cholesterol, both of which tend to raise the level of total blood lipids. Regularly eating tuna, mackerel, salmon, and other cold-water fish can also be beneficial.

CHANGING HABITS

The following tips may help with changing your eating habits.

▶ *If you slip and over-indulge, forgive yourself!*

▶ *The longer you stick to a healthier diet, the less likely you will have or give in to cravings.*

▶ *If you are craving a snack, eat something healthy (see page 49).*

▶ *Get rid of temptation by removing unhealthful foods from your refrigerator and cupboard.*

▶ *Enlist the support of family members and friends. If they are eating tempting foods in front of you, it will make sticking to your plan more difficult.*

WATCH YOUR WEIGHT Monitoring your weight and keeping it at a healthy level is very important when you are recovering from a heart attack or heart surgery.

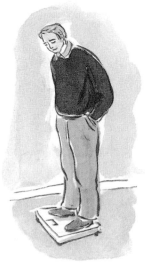

Feldenkrais Method

Living with heart disease often makes people fearful of exercise or even of moving around. By helping you learn to move with "a minimum of effort and a maximum of efficiency," the Feldenkrais Method can relieve this fear.

Origins

Born in Russia, Moshe Feldenkrais (1904–1984), a physicist, settled in Israel in the 1950s. He developed his method of movement after suffering a severe sports injury to his knee. Instead of having surgery as recommended by his doctor, he resolved to cure himself and was eventually able to walk without pain. He taught his method to friends and family members and succeeded in relieving their aches and pains. He then set up the Feldenkrais Institute in Tel Aviv.

Among his most famous students were Israel's first prime minister, David Ben-Gurion, and the violinist Yehudi Menuhin. His book, *Awareness Through Movement* (1972), made his teaching available throughout the rest of the world.

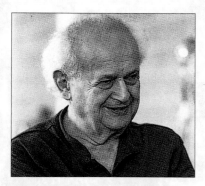

AWARENESS THROUGH MOVEMENT
Moshe Feldenkrais developed a method of gentle movement that is practiced all over the world.

A method of awareness through movement, consisting of a series of gentle movements explored under the guidance of a teacher, the Feldenkrais Method can help you correct poor physical habits that put undo strain on your joints and muscles. You are encouraged to become aware of how your muscles and joints feel, so that you can learn how to move in ways that will not cause damage.

How can the Feldenkrais Method help me after a heart attack?

The gentle movements performed during a lesson will help you feel at ease with your body. Heart patients have often lost this feeling through fear of pain—either from angina attacks or from having experienced a heart attack. If they have had surgery, they will also have suffered pain from the operation. With Feldenkrais you learn how to organize all your movements in relation to gravity, so that they become easier and more graceful. The movements taught are pleasurable and easy because Feldenkrais teachers believe that maximum learning occurs with the least amount of effort.

Can the movements be dangerous for someone with heart disease?

Any physical exertion can be harmful if it is done incorrectly or too strenuously. Feldenkrais teachers, however, make sure that students work within their own limits. The movements (teachers do not refer to them as exercises) should never cause discomfort. However, you should tell the teacher of your medical condition before the class begins. As with all activity for heart patients, you must consult your doctor before you sign up for classes.

Can the Feldenkrais Method help with pain relief?

The Feldenkrais Method does not offer direct pain relief, but it can make the movements you perform every day less painful by showing you how to move your body more harmoniously.

Particularly during one-to-one sessions, a Feldenkrais teacher will gently lead you into positions that you may have associated with pain or fear. For example, someone whose chest is painful after heart surgery can learn to move his upper body more freely by making greater use of the range of subtle movements that are possible in the neck, shoulder, spine, and ribs.

Can the Feldenkrais Method change mental attitudes?

The Feldenkrais lessons often have a profound effect on how people feel and behave. By learning to relax tense muscles, you will gradually feel more at ease. Your breathing is also likely to improve.

The lessons may have effects on an emotional level as well. Some people find that strong feelings arise during a lesson and are released when the teacher leads their body through particular movements. Although this is a fairly common effect, it is not the main focus of the method.

Can the Feldenkrais Method improve circulation?

By releasing tension and showing you how to make your muscles work with one another, the method will improve your circulation. The movements used in the lesson are too slow and gentle to be a form of aerobic exercise. But they can help to prepare you for performing more vigorous exercise, such as walking, jogging, or swimming, by teaching you to move in such a way that you do not put your body under unnecessary stress.

How long will it take before I notice an improvement?

Many people feel much better and more at ease after the first lesson. To change a lifetime of bad habits takes longer. A course of 6 to 12 lessons is average, although some people take occasional lessons for years to keep from sliding back into bad habits. Feldenkrais himself suggested one lesson for every year you have lived.

What happens during a lesson?

There are two types of lessons—one-to-one sessions and group lessons. The group lesson, Awareness through Movement, lasts 45 to 60 minutes. Classes are usually small, although Feldenkrais on occasion taught 100 students at a time.

Most lessons start with students in a resting position. The teacher then guides you through a sequence of movements and talks you through various positions. You are asked to pay attention to how movements feel by actively listening to your body. Both beginners and experienced students can attend the same class.

During the one-to-one sessions, known as Functional Integration, the teacher will guide you with gentle touch through a series of movements. You may be asked to lie on a low padded table, to sit on a chair, or even to stand in a comfortable position, while the teacher explores various patterns of movement with you and asks occasional questions designed to stimulate your awareness.

Which type of lesson should I take?

One-to-one lessons are good for heart patients because the teacher can help you overcome specific problems you face. These lessons, however, are more expensive. Group sessions are also beneficial, but you should tell your teacher about your condition.

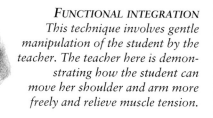

FUNCTIONAL INTEGRATION
This technique involves gentle manipulation of the student by the teacher. The teacher here is demonstrating how the student can move her shoulder and arm more freely and relieve muscle tension.

Students can benefit equally from both kinds of lessons because they complement each other.

How are Feldenkrais teachers trained?

Qualified teachers complete 800 hours of training over a four-year period. You can find a teacher by contacting the Feldenkrais Guild in Albany, Oregon. For French-speaking practitioners, get in touch with the Feldendrais Institute of Somatic Education, Inc., in Montreal, Canada. If there isn't a Feldenkrais teacher in your area, these groups can tell you where to buy audio tapes that will guide you through the lessons.

WHAT YOU CAN DO AT HOME

This sequence of movements will help you explore how you feel as you move. The point is not to do it right but to pay attention to how you feel.

1. Sit upright on the edge of a chair, with feet flat on the floor. Turn your head to the right, as far as feels natural. Repeat four or five times. Notice how far to the right you were able to look.
2. Place your hands gently on either side of your neck so that they form a collar, with fingertips on the back of your neck and wrists meeting under your chin. Now turn your head to the right again, repeating four or five times. On the last turn, hold the pose.
3. Take your hands off your neck. See if you can now look a bit farther than you could before, again without straining.
4. Place hands on your neck again. Turn head to the right; hold. Return your gaze to the front and again to the right several times (only the eyes move); return to face the front.
5. Remove your hands and rest. Feel how easily you are breathing.
6. Now turn your head to the right again. Compare how far you can look to the right now with how far you could in Step 1. Repeat the process, this time looking to the left.

MANAGING STRESS

Stress, one of the leading causes of heart trouble, needs to be managed. You can learn to keep stress under control instead of letting it control you.

Much of the current research into the causes of heart disease points a finger at stress. It not only raises blood pressure but also elevates cholesterol levels. For example, accountants at the end of the tax year and students at exam time have both been found to have elevated cholesterol levels. Getting stress under control is a vital part of a recovery program.

Stress occurs when the situation with which a person is faced is more than he or she can cope with. It can happen dozens of times a day and be brought on by little annoyances, like the phone ringing while you are in the shower, or a major life crisis, such as a diagnosis of heart disease.

PHYSICAL EFFECTS OF STRESS

Stress causes physical reactions known as the fight-or-flight response. When you are faced with a stressful situation, your body prepares for action: Your heart beats faster, your coronary arteries constrict, and your body's energy supply system—the blood—moves into overdrive, flowing away from nonessential organs like the stomach to the muscles. Preparing for possible injury, your blood clots more quickly.

Although the changes brought on by stress are essential for running away from or facing up to danger, none of them is desirable in a person who has heart disease. If stress and the reactions to it occurred only once in a while, there would be no problem; your body would simply return to normal. But often stress occurs many times a day, keeping individuals in chronic states of anxiety.

The risks to your heart

If you have heart disease, your body is at greater risk for being damaged by stress. This happens because narrowed and damaged coronary arteries are hyper-responsive to stress hormones, which cause the arteries to constrict, even go into spasm. The results are higher blood pressure and increased clotting possibilities, which make the existing problems even worse.

Although stress does hit heart patients harder, you should not stop working or take to your bed in an attempt to avoid it—boredom can also be stressful—but you do need to learn to handle stressful situations more effectively. Ideally you should respond to challenges or difficult situations fast and efficiently and then relax.

STRESS AND YOUR HEART

When you become stressed, production of the hormones adrenaline and cortisol increases to prepare your body to cope with the anticipated threat, even if it is only a psychological rather than a physical one. These hormones speed up the heart and increase the stickiness of blood platelets, making the blood clot more easily, and they increase the production of cholesterol and other fats such as triglycerides.

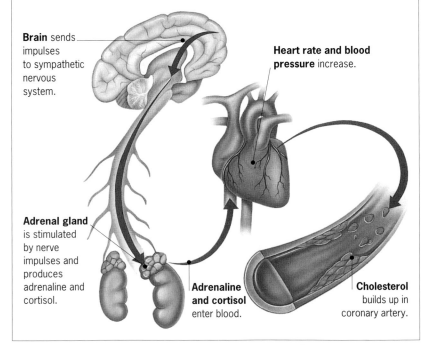

Brain sends impulses to sympathetic nervous system.

Heart rate and blood pressure increase.

Adrenal gland is stimulated by nerve impulses and produces adrenaline and cortisol.

Adrenaline and cortisol enter blood.

Cholesterol builds up in coronary artery.

Many therapies can help you get more in touch with your inner feelings and emotions and respond better to life's challenges. Counseling and support groups can be especially valuable. One-to-one counseling can provide you with a safe place to discuss your worries—about returning to work after a heart attack, for example, or coping with the stresses of life—and a support group can help you realize that you are not alone in your battle to recover. Members of a group might, for instance, help each other stick to a low-fat, heart-healthy way of eating. They could also provide emotional support. Many cardiac rehabilitation centers include support groups in their programs.

Art, dance, and music therapy are all geared to helping people understand themselves better. Under the supervision of a trained therapist, you can paint or draw, dance, or play music as a way of expressing how you feel about your body, your life, and your heart.

COPING WITH STRESS
Some people seem to be able to handle stress much better than others; they rarely become bothered by traffic jams, long lines, noisy neighbors, or distressing news stories.

What protects some people from stress may simply be a question of personality; they are naturally more laid back than others. Many people who are more easygoing and seldom get angry also have a high sense of self-esteem, according to many studies. Hostile people tend to have lower self-esteem. Improving your self-esteem may be a means of making you more relaxed and improving your health. The more you think you are worth, the more likely you are to do things that preserve your health, such as eating sensibly, exercising regularly, and keeping your stress levels as low as possible.

A new way of living and working
Realizing that they have had a brush with death, many people who have had a heart attack or major heart surgery find themselves reviewing their lives. Some of the things that used to seem so important—meeting a sales target or keeping up with neighbors, for example—suddenly become less significant. Reassessing your priorities is one of the things that makes stress management easier to learn. When you realize that keeping healthy and enjoying life are your major priorities, it is easier to put everything else into perspective.

The benefits of support
One factor that can help protect against the negative effects of stress is having a good social network. This doesn't necessarily mean knowing influential people or having dozens of acquaintances. It means feeling connected with family, friends, and your community. A study of more than 13,000 people in Finland found that people who were socially isolated were two or three times more likely to die of heart disease and all other causes. Even just being a member of a club or religious organization decreased the risk of early death.

Social isolation is believed to be as significant a factor in death rates as smoking, high blood pressure, high cholesterol, obesity, and lack of physical exercise. Being a part of your community and becoming more involved with friends and family may also help you to regain your health.

A study at Yale University Medical School of 1,192 healthy people 50 to 79 years of age showed that those with partners and strong family ties had lower levels of the hormones noradrenaline and cortisol. Both are believed to influence blood pressure and the heart's response to stress, confirming that emotional support helps your heart.

MANAGING STRESSFUL SITUATIONS
The best way to deal with stressful situations is either to avoid them in the first place or not let them bother you. With planning, you can arrange your life so that you experience less stress. If you find that seeing a particular friend or relative makes you tense, either stop seeing that person or, if this is not possible, choose to see the person less often or for a limited amount of time. If you find certain chores burdensome, reward yourself with a swim, a massage, a walk in the park, or a funny video when you have completed them. If someone is doing something that really annoys you, either decide

Learn to laugh
Whenever you laugh, your body releases chemicals called endorphins, which have an action similar to that of morphine—they make you feel good. If you find something to laugh about every day, you will be better able to cope with life's challenges.

A good way to unwind in the evening is to watch something funny on television. You can videotape comedy programs and save them to watch later or rent funny films. Humorous books and cartoons and cassette tapes of old comedy radio programs are other good ways to lighten your life with laughter.

*SOCIALIZING FOR YOUR HEART
Getting together regularly with friends and feeling connected with people in your community can reduce your risk of dying from heart disease.*

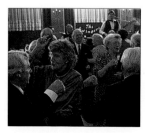

that it is not worth being annoyed about or let the annoying person know how you feel by telling him or her calmly what bothers you about such behavior.

If you can't change a situation, then learn not to let it get you down. Remember, you are in control of how you feel. You can choose to let certain things make you angry or not. It can help to change the channels in your mind and think about something else; plan a holiday in the sun, for instance, or think other pleasant thoughts.

Meditating, deep breathing, progressive muscle relaxation, yoga, and aerobic exercise can make stress easier to handle. They decrease your physical reactions to stress and help your body get back to normal faster after the fight-or-flight reaction has kicked into action. Deep breathing can be particularly useful because you can do it anywhere—at work, standing in a supermarket line, or waiting in traffic for a red light to change to green.

Having a massage once a week, either from a friend or a professional massage therapist, is another way to relieve stress. It provides deep relaxation. If you have a massage with scented oils, a form of aromatherapy, you can achieve additional benefits. The massage therapist can choose oils to lift your mood and give you extra energy or to relax you and help you sleep better.

LEARNING TO MANAGE TIME
A lot of stress comes from not having enough time to do everything that needs to be done. You can't make the day longer, but you can make better use of the time you have. When you are not in a hurry, you will feel more relaxed and in control of your life. Leave early for work and other appointments, so that unexpected delays won't make you late (and anxious). Carry a book with you, so you will have something to do while waiting in line at the bank; then you won't feel you are wasting time.

RELAXING AT THE OFFICE

The workplace is often a major source of physical tension. Your neck may feel stiff, your shoulders knotty and painful, and your back achy from sitting too long, attending stressful meetings, and putting in long hours. These stretches, which can be done at your desk and take only a few minutes, can provide great relief.

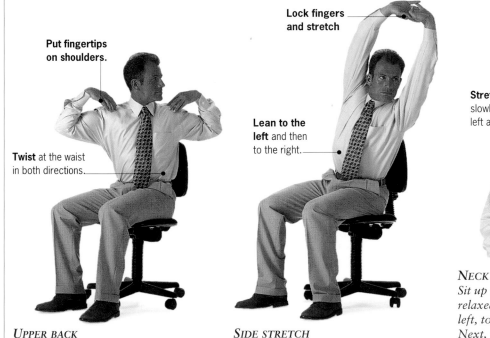

Put fingertips on shoulders.

Twist at the waist in both directions.

Lock fingers and stretch

Lean to the left and then to the right.

Stretch neck slowly to the left and the right.

UPPER BACK
Place hands on your shoulders, then twist at the waist until you feel a stretch across your upper back. Repeat in the other direction.

SIDE STRETCH
Shrug shoulders up and down until they are relaxed. Lock fingers with palms facing upward. Stretch up as high as you can, then lean over to each side.

NECK
Sit up straight but keep your body relaxed. Slowly drop your neck to the left, to the right, and then to your chest. Next, roll your head all the way to the left, then back to the center, and, finally, all the way to the right. Do not roll your head backward because this puts dangerous pressure on your neck.

Returning to work

Most people can go back to the jobs they were doing before their heart attack or bypass surgery. In fact, working can help you maintain your self-esteem and keep you involved with society. But working can also be a source of stress. You should go back to work equipped with a new attitude because stress on the job may have contributed to your illness in the first place.

Use time management skills to help you get everything done. Get up a little earlier, so that you don't need to start off in a rush. Arrive at the office a few minutes early and sit down to organize your day. By setting priorities and planning your work day accordingly, you can save time and avoid last-minute panics.

Timing helps

One way to see how well you are managing your time is to keep a diary; jot down everything you do in a day for a week or so. Then review it to see if there are any tasks you can trim down, cut out, or combine. Allocate your time to specific tasks. Break bigger tasks into stages. Tackling jobs step-by-step makes them less daunting and in the process, you may even discover some shortcuts that get them done more efficiently.

Take it easy

You should also decide that you are going to take things a little easier at work. This does not mean becoming known as the lazy one. It does mean not overcommitting yourself. Refuse to be a perfectionist—learn to do a good enough job. To keep your workload at a manageable level, never volunteer to do extra tasks for which you do not have ample time available and delegate as many tasks as you can. At first you may find it hard to delegate. You may feel that you are the only person who can get things done properly, but if you make yourself ill you won't get it done at all.

When faced with an unpleasant or difficult task, take a few minutes to prepare yourself. Breathe deeply, shut your eyes for a moment, or stretch at your desk. Most importantly, don't simply put it off or forget to do it. The problem probably won't go away and when it comes up again, it will have become more urgent or more out of hand, making your life even more stressful than if you had taken prompt action.

ART FOR YOUR HEART

Art therapy is now offered in many hospitals as an adjunct to counseling to deal with the psychological effects of illness. After heart surgery, many patients find painting very relaxing; at the same time it helps them express hidden feelings. Patients are encouraged to draw their feelings, a process that often enables them to express fears and anxieties they could not verbalize. Art therapy has proved to be very valuable to heart patients, who may experience strong feelings of

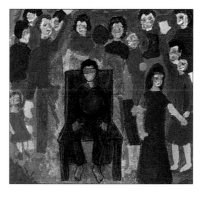

depression after cardiac surgery. Drawings are sometimes literal, showing the person feeling depressed, or perhaps angry at the doctor, but they are very often symbolic, revealing thoughts that were pushed away because they were too painful to deal with.

A trained art therapist will analyze a patient's drawings, interpreting the color, choice of subject, and placement of objects in the picture (pictures often depict recurrent dreams, which also provide a clue to feelings). The therapist may make recommendations for subsequent drawings, in order to draw out other feelings.

ART THERAPY
This painting was done by a heart-surgery patient who felt that he was excluded from joining his friends' activity. The blindfold represents his feeling of isolation from those around him.

Leave work at work

When the work day ends—stop working! You should leave your work behind you not only physically but mentally as well. If at all possible, do not take work home with you and make a concerted effort not to worry about the job while you are at home or out trying to enjoy leisure activities.

It is especially important for individuals suffering from heart disease to unwind at the end of the day. Before you go home, take a walk round the block or through a park. When you arrive home, change out of your work clothes into an at-home outfit to reinforce the demarcation between your work life and home life and help you to feel more relaxed.

Join a health club and, after your doctor has given you the go-ahead, go for a workout or a swim after work, or just drop in to relax in the spa bath. Exercise is a proven method of releasing tension and is especially beneficial when it is done regularly. It is also good for strengthening your heart.

Stress Reduction

It is vital for survivors of heart attacks or heart surgery and anyone with a diagnosed heart problem or hypertension to reduce their stress levels. Dancing is a fun and effective way to release negative feelings, and yoga routines are calming.

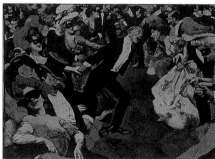

DANCING
Throughout the ages various types of dancing have been used as a means of relaxation and also as a way to express feelings. This 1911 painting of a masked ball shows one of the forms it can take.

Stress has many causes, and it may be hard to eliminate them. For instance, what can you do about irritating colleagues or friends who are always late for appointments? The answer is to release the tension.

Stress responses are often learned at an early age, and by adulthood habitual responses to stress are likely to be ingrained. But even impatient, competitive people can change their responses to stressful situations with dance therapy and yoga. Regular practice of these techniques can have long-lasting benefits to the health of body and mind, and are particularly applicable to attaining a healthier heart. As beneficial as they are, however, you should check with your doctor before doing these exercises.

DANCING OUT YOUR NEGATIVITY

Dance is a universal expression of human emotions, and 30 minutes of directed dancing can bring peace and relief from tension. Try the following formula for releasing a specific negative emotion.

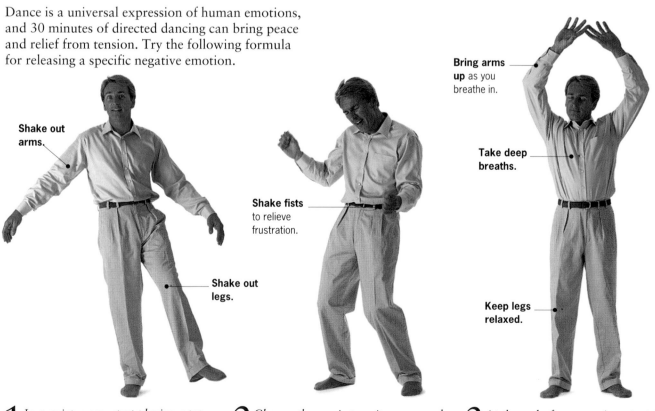

Shake out arms.

Shake out legs.

Shake fists to relieve frustration.

Bring arms up as you breathe in.

Take deep breaths.

Keep legs relaxed.

1 *In a quiet room, start playing a tape of soft music to relax and get into the mood. Swing your body freely with floppy arms and legs, shaking them out.*

2 *Change the music to suit your mood, then just express yourself physically, depending on your feelings. Stamp and shout or move slowly.*

3 *At the end of your session, start to wind down and relax, letting go of your emotions with a few deep, slow breaths. Then sit quietly for a while.*

YOGA

Yoga is an ideal way to wind down from stress. Try the following two routines on a daily basis for a month and notice how relaxed you feel.

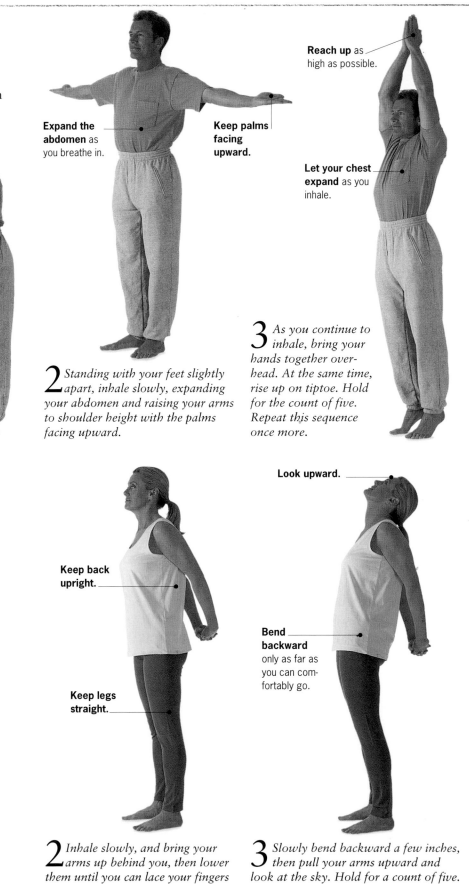

Drop head to chest.

Relax shoulders.

1 *Exhale deeply, relaxing your shoulders and chest and contracting your abdomen. At the same time, let your body go limp, with your head and arms hanging downward and your palms facing your body.*

Expand the abdomen as you breathe in.

Keep palms facing upward.

2 *Standing with your feet slightly apart, inhale slowly, expanding your abdomen and raising your arms to shoulder height with the palms facing upward.*

Reach up as high as possible.

Let your chest expand as you inhale.

3 *As you continue to inhale, bring your hands together overhead. At the same time, rise up on tiptoe. Hold for the count of five. Repeat this sequence once more.*

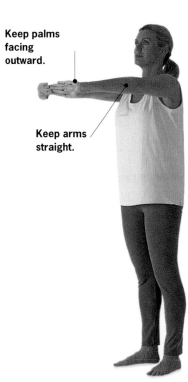

Keep palms facing outward.

Keep arms straight.

1 *Stand straight and raise your hands to touch your chest, with palms facing outward and fingers touching. Straighten your arms in front of you, feeling the elbows stretch.*

Keep back upright.

Keep legs straight.

2 *Inhale slowly, and bring your arms up behind you, then lower them until you can lace your fingers together, keeping your back straight and your head up.*

Look upward.

Bend backward only as far as you can comfortably go.

3 *Slowly bend backward a few inches, then pull your arms upward and look at the sky. Hold for a count of five. Exhale, then relax. Repeat this sequence once more.*

CONTROLLING ANGER AND HOSTILITY

Anger and hostility can put you at great risk for developing heart disease. Learning to control these negative emotions will not only reduce the risk but will also help you enjoy life more.

Two distinct personality types, A and B, were first described in the 1950s by two American cardiologists, Meyer Friedman and Ray Rosenman (see page 32). Since then, many studies have looked at the effects of personality on heart disease, and both anger and hostility have been identified as major risk factors.

The Western Collaborative Group Study, which began in the 1970s, followed 3,154 healthy California men over nearly nine years to see which of them would develop heart disease. Each had filled in a questionnaire designed to reveal characteristics of personality. The study found that of those patients who did develop heart disease (336), all had one thing in common—they had answered seven questions, designed to evaluate whether or not they were hostile, in a way that indicated a high level of hostility. Subsequent studies also showed that the people who scored high on the anger and hostility sections of personality tests were more likely to develop heart disease. Thus, hostility seems to be an important link between personality and heart disease, along with how a person reacts to stress.

HOW ANGER HURTS YOUR HEART

Anger, hostility, and aggression increase the risk of heart disease in several ways. They all cause blood pressure to rise. Several studies have also shown that the blood pressure of people who are often angry goes up faster and stays up longer.

Anger also makes the body produce more adrenaline and cortisol, which increase the amount of fat in the blood, and more noradrenaline, which makes the blood's platelets stickier. The increased fat is often deposited in the lining of the arteries, where it forms plaques, while the sticky platelets tend to form clots more easily. As the clots attempt to move through the arteries that are narrowed by plaques, they get stuck and obstruct blood flow. When this happens in the heart, you have a heart attack; in the brain, a stroke.

People who are hostile may be more likely to smoke, drink alcohol to excess, and overeat, possibly as a way of relieving the tension caused by their anger. All these habits increase the risk of heart disease.

Some researchers have found that angry people tend to be more socially isolated as well; they don't trust others enough to make friends easily. Social isolation has been shown in study after study to impede recovery from illness and contribute to death from heart disease.

Anger after heart disease

If being an angry person can lead to heart problems, it also has the potential to cause even more damage to a heart already weakened by disease. To make matters worse, once you know how damaging anger is to your heart, you may find yourself getting even angrier because of the "unfairness" of the situation. But you can learn to control your anger instead of letting it control you.

MANAGING ANGER

The key to protecting yourself from the harmful effects of hostility is learning to control it. At one time people believed that the best thing to do with anger was express it. Suppressing anger, it was thought, could be emotionally and perhaps even physically harmful. Current research suggests that the best strategy for dealing with anger is to

continued on page 155

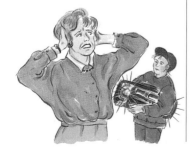

ANGER-GENERATING SITUATIONS
A teenager playing loud music is only one of the situations that might make you feel angry without even realizing it. It is important to recognize anger and then to deal with it appropriately. In this case, ask the teenager to turn down the music or put plugs in your ears.

ARE YOU EASILY ANGERED?

If you spend your life feeling irritated or have frequent bursts of anger, then you are a likely candidate for high blood pressure, which will put you at risk for heart disease. At one time, releasing anger was viewed as acceptable therapy for many emotional problems. Now the view is that it is best not to get angry, but rather to control yourself and express your feelings in a constructive way. You can take this quiz to find out how angry you get at everyday situations.

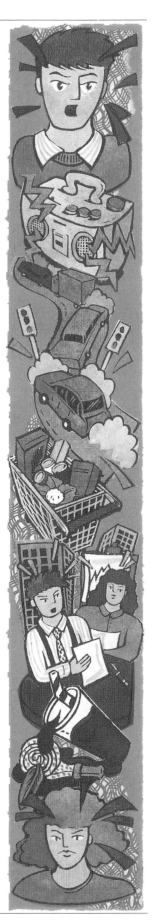

YOUR NEIGHBORS REGULARLY PLAY MUSIC VERY LOUDLY. DO YOU

a) Politely ask them to restrict the noise levels after certain hours?
b) Turn up your own stereo or television fully and hammer on the wall until they get the hint?

YOUR NORMAL ROUTE TO WORK IS DISRUPTED BECAUSE OF LOCAL ROAD WORK. DO YOU

a) Reroute your journeys for the next few days?
b) Telephone the city council from your car phone and shout at the receptionist about the situation?

YOU ARE STUCK IN RUSH HOUR TRAFFIC. DO YOU

a) Spend the time preparing your thoughts for the day ahead or plans for the evening?
b) Pull up as close as possible to the car in front and rev your engine?

SOMEONE WRONGLY ACCUSES YOU OF A MINOR MISTAKE. DO YOU

a) Calmly explain that there must be a misunderstanding?
b) Seethe about it for hours and later verbally attack the accuser?

THE SUPERMARKET LINE IS REALLY LONG AND THE CHECKOUT PERSON IS VERY SLOW. DO YOU

a) Realize that being impatient will not speed your journey to the front of the line?
b) Glare at the people in front of you and comment loudly on the store's lack of organization?

A FAMILY MEMBER CRITICIZES SOMETHING YOU HAVE DONE. DO YOU

a) Consider the points that have been raised to see if they are valid?
b) Take it as an intentional personal attack?

WHAT DO YOU THINK OF THE PHRASE "LIFE IS FULL OF LITTLE ANNOYANCES?"

a) It's true, but most of the time they can be overcome.
b) It's true, and they make my life 10 times harder.

IN A MEETING AT WORK, ONE OF YOUR COLLEAGUES FORCEFULLY DISAGREES WITH YOU. DO YOU

a) Agree to differ—after all, everyone has their own opinions?
b) Shout down your colleague, then leave the meeting?

A FRIEND BEHAVES BADLY AT YOUR PARTY. DO YOU

a) Ignore it and avoid him?
b) Tell him that his behavior is unacceptable and ask him to leave?

YOU CONTROL YOUR ANGER DURING THE DAY. DO YOU FIND THAT THIS

a) Stops you from overreacting.
b) Makes you so angry that you randomly explode over something that is quite minor?

HOW ANGRY ARE YOU?
If you answered mostly a's, you have learned to curb your anger, annoyance, and aggression because you can differentiate between what is serious and important and what needs to be viewed with a more tolerant perspective. This, however, does not mean you aren't assertive when assertion is needed; rather, you know how to judge when such expressions are required. This will ensure that you keep your blood pressure at a healthy, even level.

   If you answered mostly b's, you are set off by life's small irritations quite randomly and unjustifiably. This indicates that you have a high level of hostility and a low level of self-confidence, not to mention a blood pressure reading that goes up and down like a yo-yo. You must work on coming to terms with your feelings and gain more self-control. You will like yourself better, and other people will find you much more approachable.

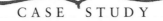
An Angry Man

Constant hostility toward other people and the world in general is one of the greatest personality-related risk factors of heart disease. Anger raises blood pressure and cholesterol levels. Also, by making relationships with others difficult, it deprives people who become ill of the social support that they need to get well.

Mark is 45 and the owner of several successful restaurants. He is married and has two teenage children. Mark is proud of his achievements and knows they are due in part to his competitive nature. However, his temper plays a role too. About a month ago Mark suffered severe chest pains and was taken to a hospital, where he was told that he had had a mild heart attack. He returned to work after the attack as though nothing had happened, but soon found that his rages brought back his chest pain. He went to see his doctor, who prescribed some medication to relieve the pain. She also told him that to heal his heart he would have to make important changes in his life, including learning to control anger.

WHAT SHOULD MARK DO?

Mark must come to terms with both his heart attack and the factors that led to it, and the sooner he does this the better for the health of his heart. For the sake of his health he must learn to control his anger and stress levels. Diffusing potentially angry situations before they erupt is essential for preventing strain on his heart. Mark can better deal with work problems by first of all instituting more efficient procedures, communicating calmly with his staff and placing more trust in them, and improving his own management skills. He also needs to find ways to communicate with his family more effectively and without anger. It may help for him to attend a course in anger management.

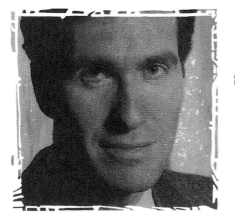

HEALTH
People with an angry and competitive personality can cause serious damage to their health.

WORK
Work can be a source of stress, and coping mechanisms are important to avoid difficult situations and confrontations.

FAMILY
Family members often don't know how to deal with an angry person in the family; they either give in to the person too much or fight back, and matters just get worse.

Action Plan

HEALTH
Attend anger-control classes and practice relaxation techniques. Exercise more to burn off stress and feelings of hostility.

WORK
Set up more efficient procedures. Learn better management skills. Hire an assistant manager to relieve pressure. Delegate more to junior staff.

FAMILY
Ask family to support attempts to control anger and be more forgiving during lapses. Spend more relaxation time with them.

HOW THINGS TURNED OUT FOR MARK

Mark acknowledged his anger problem and began to use the behavior modification techniques and relaxation exercises he learned at the coronary care unit. Despite some setbacks, which he refused to let get in the way of his recovery, his relationship with his family and staff improved. Although Mark has suffered occasional chest pains, he has been lucky so far and has not had another heart attack. He now feels more in control of his life.

ANGER-DEFUSING EXERCISE

Anger is one of the most persistent and destructive of the negative emotions. The following routine is often taught in autogenic training classes (see page 42) to deal with anger. Practice it any time you feel angry.

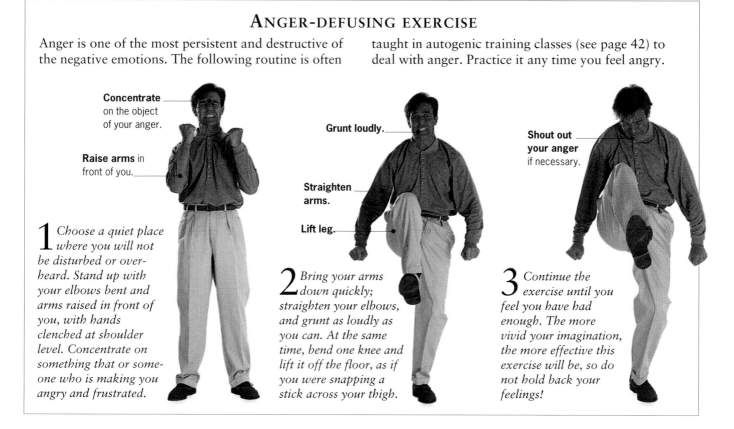

Concentrate on the object of your anger.

Raise arms in front of you.

1 *Choose a quiet place where you will not be disturbed or overheard. Stand up with your elbows bent and arms raised in front of you, with hands clenched at shoulder level. Concentrate on something that or someone who is making you angry and frustrated.*

Grunt loudly.

Straighten arms.

Lift leg.

2 *Bring your arms down quickly; straighten your elbows, and grunt as loudly as you can. At the same time, bend one knee and lift it off the floor, as if you were snapping a stick across your thigh.*

Shout out your anger if necessary.

3 *Continue the exercise until you feel you have had enough. The more vivid your imagination, the more effective this exercise will be, so do not hold back your feelings!*

neither express it nor suppress it, but to avoid feeling it, if possible. People who are not easily roused to anger are healthier and less likely to suffer heart disease than those with similar lifestyles who get angry easily. People who are angry almost all the time are most at risk of heart disease. And while it may prove difficult, they are the ones who, for the sake of their health, most need to learn to control their anger.

Defusing hostility

If you are a person who is always angry, you can learn to short-circuit your anger as soon as it starts. Specialists advise spending 20 minutes every day learning how to behave in a less hostile way. Just as your angry outlook was not formed overnight, change may not come quickly. You will have to work on curbing your anger over a long period. But the effort will be worth it. Changing your behavior could not only save your life but also make it more pleasant.

Keep a diary

The first step is to record how often you become angry, what situations trigger your rage, and how you feel afterward. Once you know what makes you angry, the next step is to learn to control your feelings. To do this, you have to recognize that you are often angry and admit that your anger is frequently inappropriate. The questionnaire on page 153 will help you identify situations in which you get angry. Record these in your diary and write down alternative ways of dealing with them. This will serve as a useful reminder for what kinds of situations to watch out for and how to handle them.

You will need to decide whether your anger is really justified. Chronically hostile people almost always believe that they are right to feel angry, so that changing this belief is an important first step.

Change your anger

After realizing that you are angry, the goal is to change your mood. There are several strategies that can help. First of all, you can reason with yourself. For example, you can tell yourself that there is no need to feel angry because the waiter brought the wrong order. Everyone makes mistakes and this one can be easily rectified. Putting things in perspective is important for reasoning away anger. Most anger-generating situations are really not worth getting worked up about, and they usually pass quickly anyway.

DIFFUSING ANGER

Anger should be diffused as soon as possible. Try some of these methods as soon as you feel angry thoughts beginning:

▶ *Count to 10 silently before you speak or act.*

▶ *Think about something pleasant, like a party you will be going to or a vacation.*

▶ *Leave the situation if possible; walk outside for a few minutes.*

▶ *Take several deep, slow breaths.*

▶ *Tell yourself that the situation is not worth getting angry about.*

▶ *Write a letter to the object of your anger, then burn it.*

Stop your thoughts

If you can't reason anger away, you can try to stop it. Simply ordering yourself to stop thinking in an angry or hostile way can be suprisingly effective. You can either silently tell yourself to stop, or you can, if you are alone, shout "Stop!"

Another method that can be used to stop angry thoughts is to think about something else. This works because you can't think about two things at once. Decide in advance what positive thoughts or situations you will turn to when something makes you angry; some people think about a delicious dinner, a funny film, or making love. Then, when you feel angry, instead of dwelling on the event that has annoyed you, turn your thoughts to the pleasant distraction that you have prepared for yourself.

Learning to meditate (see page 36) is another method that will help you feel less hostile. By meditating, you will short-circuit your body's reactions to your anger. Instead of instantly switching into overdrive, with a pounding heart, increased adrenaline, and raised blood pressure, you can learn to shift into low gear. You will have to learn a meditation technique and practice it every day in order to use this method of blocking angry feelings. Then, when you feel angry, meditate for a few moments until you feel much calmer and more in control. Not only will it take your mind off your anger but it will also switch off the physical reactions that are so damaging to your heart.

A CHANGE FOR THE BETTER

Hostile people are usually very suspicious of others. They cherish a world view in which other people are out to get them and are against them. These beliefs are self-perpetuating. If you act as if the world is against you, then it will be.

Studies have shown that hostile people have poorer social relationships than others. Some research has proved also that people who have no close relationships are less likely to survive heart disease. By developing better relationships, heart patients can improve their network of social support.

In a book called *Anger Kills,* published in the United States, Dr. Redford Williams and Dr. Virginia Williams propose a number of strategies to make the angry person more caring and trusting. They recommend learning to listen to others and becoming more empathetic, tolerant and forgiving. To improve personal relationships, they advise keeping a pet, becoming involved in your community by doing volunteer work, and finding a confidante.

Angry people also tend to be cynical about the motives of other people. This cynicism can be overcome by adopting a more positive attitude. Learning to laugh at yourself can often prevent you from getting angry at others. The Williamses also suggest looking beyond ordinary daily situations or trying to view them from a balanced perspective. They believe, too, that becoming more spiritual will help you develop a more positive mental attitude.

THE LAST DAY

One strategy is to pretend that today is your last day. If you have survived a heart attack or have to live with heart disease, you have probably used this technique without realizing it. If today were your last day on earth, would you want to waste it yelling at the dry cleaner for failing to have your clothes ready on time, or swearing at the driver who cut across your lane, or complaining about your neighbors? Wouldn't you rather spend it telling your loved ones how much they mean to you or simply enjoying every moment of the day?

ASSERTING YOURSELF

Sometimes you will find that your anger is justified. Perhaps your boss is criticizing your work, imposing impossible deadlines, and generally making your life miserable. Instead of suffering in silence or blowing up, you can make your boss aware of how you feel by asserting yourself.

Assertion means telling someone else, in a reasonable and calm way, how his or her behavior makes you feel, and then discussing how to resolve the issue. Unlike anger, it allows you to express a grievance without getting out of control. Other people are more likely to respond positively to assertive behavior than to an aggressive approach. You can probably get what you want without raising either your voice or your blood pressure.

INDEX

A

Acupressure 101
  for angina 112
  for anxiety 115
  for depression 133
  for hypertension 125
Acupuncture 101
  and quitting smoking 35
  and moxibustion 101
Age
  and arteries 26
  and blood pressure 26
  and heart disease 26, 32
Alcohol 39, 51
  and cholesterol 57, 64
  and congenital disorders 106
  and the French diet 57
  and the heart 64
  and heart muscle disease 118,
    119
  for heart patients 133
  and high blood pressure 51
  and the Mediterranean diet 56
  safe levels of 64
  and triglycerides 53
Aneurysm
  aortic 129
  and blood pressure 129
  brain (berry) 129
Anger
  control of 152, 154
  diffusing 156
    exercise for 155
  and heart disease 152
  questionnaire 153
  self-assertion 156
  social relationships 156
Angina 77, 86
  and atherosclerosis 108
  and exercise 86
  first aid for 86
  and heart disease 110
  herbs for 102
Angiography 98
Angioplasty 111
  and heart attacks 113
  for intermittent claudication
    129
Antioxidants 58
  and atherosclerosis 58
  bioflavonoids 59
  and blood clotting 127
  and French diet 57
  Mediterranean diet 56
  and vegetarians 58
Aromatherapy 100
  for atherosclerosis 110
  for depression 133
  inhalation 101

Arrhythmias 114
  atrial fibrillation 87
  bradycardia 88, 114
  defibrillator 115
  and heart attacks 114
  pacemakers 115
  tachycardia 88, 114
  see also Palpitations
Arteries 16
  and age 26
  and blood pressure 22
  coronary 19, 21
  diseased 110
  herbs for 110
  see also Atherosclerosis
Art therapy 149
Aspirin 114
  and heart attacks 113
Atheromas 108
Atherosclerosis (hardening of
    arteries) 25, 108
  and age 26
  and plaques 52, 108
  and women 108
Autogenic training 42

B

Barnard, Christiaan 120
Biofeedback 104
  and blood pressure 141
Bioflavonoids 59
Blood
  circulation of 16
  deoxygenated 16
  oxygenated 16
  red blood cells 17
  tests 90
  vessels 17
Blood clots 126
  and anticoagulants 126
  and aspirin 114
  and atherosclerosis 108
  herbs for 102
  and stress 146
  test for clotting 91
  see also Thrombosis
Blood pressure
  and age 24, 26
  and alcohol 51, 64
  and arteries 22
  and caffeine 64
  and contraceptive pill 46
  controlling 22, 41, 140
  and coronary heart disease 41
  diastolic 22, 40
  and dietary changes 51, 141
  and exercise 141
  herbs for 102

high and low 22
  maintaining normal 23
  measuring 23, 25, 41, 46, 96
  and minerals 51, 125, 141
  normal 23
  and obesity 51
  pet therapy 140
  during pregnancy 25, 41
  reducing 25, 140
  risk factors 23
  and salt 51
  and stress 140, 146
  systolic 22, 40
  variations in 40
  see also Hypertension
Blood vessels 17
  herbs for 102
  see also Arteries
Blue babies 107
Breathlessness 86, 88

C

Caffeine
  and blood pressure 64
  effects on heart 64
  for heart patients 133
Calcium
  to lower blood pressure 141
Capillary network 17
Cardiac rehabilitation
  exercises 136
  phases of 136
  Rehabilitation Manager 138
Cardiomyopathy 118
  heart transplant 119
Cardiopulmonary resuscitation
    (CPR) 116
Carbohydrates 49, 56
Catheterization 95, 111
  angiography 98
  angioplasty 111
  balloon flotation 95
  blood pressure 95
  electrode 95
  and embolism 126
  in fetus 108
  shaving 111
  and thrombosis 126
  valvuloplasty 118
  venography 98
Checkups 44
  physical examination 90
Chest pain 44, 86
  and heart attack 113
Cholesterol 38, 48
  and alcohol 57, 64
  and antioxidants 58
  and family history 32

and fiber 60
  and garlic 61
  herbs for 102
  high-density lipoprotein
    (HDL) 38, 52
  low-density lipoprotein (LDL)
    38, 52
  and obesity 51
  reducing 39, 143
  risks of high 39
  and saturated fat 57
  and stress 146
  testing 46, 52, 96
  transport in body 38
Circulatory system 16
  and acupuncture 101
  fetal 24
  herbs for 102
  hydrotherapy for 99
Coffee
  and cholesterol 64
  see also Caffeine
Congenital heart disorders 20,
    24, 26, 106
  atria and ventricles 107
  and breastfeeding 107
  hole in the heart 106, 109
  patent ductus arteriosus 106
  tetralogy of fallot 107
  transposition of arteries 106
  valve disorders 107
Congestive heart failure 120
  and race 29
  and salt 121
Contraceptive pill
  and blood pressure testing 46
  and familial hyper-
    lipidemia 32
  and heart disease 28
  and triglycerides 53
Coronary arteries 19, 21
  cororonary artery bypass
    112, 113, 134
  diseased 110
  and fatty deposits 21
  see also Angina,
    Atherosclerosis,
    Catheterization
Coronary heart disease
  see Heart disease
Cramps 86, 88
  and exercise 88
  and intermittent
    claudication 129
CT scan 95

D

Dance therapy 150
Depression 133
   acupressure for 133
   aromatherapy for 133
Diabetes 32
   and ethnicity 32
   and fiber 61
   and heart disease 32
   and obesity 51
   and triglycerides 53
Diet
   complex carbohydrates 49
   daily calorie intake 53, 142
   for depression 133
   eating habits 49, 50, 51, 143
   fast food 49
   fat intake 48
   fiber 60
   food pyramid 62
   French diet 57
   healthy 49, 55
   for heart patients 133
   high-risk and low-risk 58
   Mediterranean diet 48, 56
   reducing fats 54
   vegetarian 58
   weekly menu 63
   see also Antioxidants, Fats,
      Food, Weight
Diuretics
   herbal 102, 118
   for swollen ankles 89
   and tachycardia 88
Dizziness 86, 87

E

Echocardiography 94
Ectopic heartbeats 88
Edema 88
Electrocardiography (ECG)
   46, 91
   holter monitoring 93
   exercise (stress test) 46, 93
Embolism 126
   cerebral 126, 128
   pulmonary 126
   and stroke 127
Endocarditis 119
   rheumatic fever 117
   and valve disorders 115
Estrogen
   and heart disease 25
   and cholesterol 29
Exercise 39
   aerobic 67, 71, 75
   anaerobic 71
   benefits of 66
   and blood pressure 70, 141
   and cardiac output 66
   caution with 67
   and cholesterol 67
   circuit training 75
   cooling down 75

   effects on body 67
   and fat burning 66
   and a heart condition 75
   and heart muscle 70
   and heart rate 66
   home equipment 76
   personal trainer 72
   and risk of heart disease 67
   sports 71
   stretching 78
   the talk test 68
   toning 80
   warming up 75
   weekly program 74
   see also Fitness

F

Fainting 86, 87
Familial hypercholesterolemia 32
Family history
   and heart disease 29
Fatigue 86, 88
   in children 107
Fats
   chemical bond 52
   and cholesterol 52
   daily calorie intake 49
   daily target 53
   in dairy products 54
   in the diet 38
   essential fatty acids 53
   fish oils 53
   and food labels 56
   and heart disease 48, 52
   hydrogenated 53
   monounsaturated 52, 53, 57
   omega-3 fatty acids 57
   polyunsaturated 52, 53, 57
   reducing 54, 55
   saturated 48, 49, 52, 57
   trans fatty acids 53
   triglycerides 53
Fiber 60
   action of 60
   and cholesterol 60–61
   and diabetes 61
   and the heart 60
   soluble and insoluble 60
   sources of 60
Framingham Study 28, 61, 82
Feldenkrais Method 144
Fitness 67
   aerobic fitness index test 69
   assessment of 67, 69
   components of 67–69
   flexibility test 69
   for heart patients 136
   maximum heart rate 70
   monitoring 70
   muscle strength test 69
   rate of perceived exertion 70
   target heart rate zone 70
   see also Exercise
Food(s)
   dairy products 54

   eggs 62
   fish 53, 110
   frozen 48
   fruits and vegetables 48, 49, 56
   garlic 61
   heart-healthy
   high-protein 55
   labels 56
   processed 51
   pyramid 62
   snacks 49
Free radicals 58

G

Garlic
   and heart disease 61
Gender
   and heart disease 25

H

Hardening of the arteries, *see*
   Atherosclerosis
Harvey, William
   and circulation 18
Heart
   in adolescence 24
   in adulthood 24
   aging 25
   anatomy 19
   aorta 19
   atria 18
   beat 20
   cardiac output 21, 25
   conduction system 20
   congenital disorders 20, 24,
      106
   effect of weight on 38
   fetal development of 24, 106
   herbs for 102
   murmurs 20, 90
   during pregnancy 25
   sounds 20, 90
   stroke volume 21, 25
   transplant 119
   valves 19
   ventricles 18
Heart attack 112
   activity after 132
   and arrhythmias 114
   and aspirin 113
   and atherosclerosis 112
   blood test for enzymes
      after 91, 113
   cardiopulmonary resuscitation
      (CPR) 116
   driving after 136
   emotional response to 133
   first aid for 89
   and fish intake 53
   and quitting smoking 137
   returning to work after 149
   sexual relations after 137
   and thrombosis 52

Heart disease
   and age 26, 32
   and anger 152
   and cholesterol 52
   death rates from 48
   and diabetes 32
   and ethnicity 29, 32
   family history of 29
   and fats 48, 52
   and gender 29
   menopause 29, 30
   and obesity 51
   and personality 32, 152
   risk factors for 28
   risk questionnaire 33
   and smoking 34
   and stress 146
   symptoms of 86
   and weight 51
Heart failure, congestive
   120
Heart muscle disease 118
   and alcohol 118, 119
   cardiomyopathy 118
   myocarditis 118
   and transplant 119
Heart rate 21
   and caffeine 64
   and exercise 70
   monitor 97
   and rhythm disorders
      114
   target heart rate zone 70
   see also Arrhythmias
Heart surgery
   coronary artery bypass 112
   depression after 133
   driving after 136
   returning to work after 149
   sexual relations after 137
Heart valve disorders 115
Herbal medicine 101
   herb chart 102
   heart tea 103
   preparations 103
   hawthorn berry infusion 103
Hole in the heart 106, 109
Homeopathy 103
   diagnosis in 91
Hormone replacement therapy
   (HRT) and heart disease 29
Hydrotherapy 99, 122
Hyperlipoproteinemia 32
Hypertension 23, 124
   avoiding 51
   effects of 41
   and race 29
   see also Blood pressure
Hypnotherapy 104
   and quitting smoking 35

I

Infections
   and congenital disorders 107
   and endocarditis 119

and heart muscle disorders
118
and pericarditis 119
and valve disorders 117, 118
Intermittent claudication 129
and atherosclerosis 108
and smoking 129
Imaging techniques 93–95
Iron overload 64

L

Lymphatic system 17
Lungs
and circulation 16
Lipids 48, 91
blood tests for 91
see also Fats
Luthe, Wolfgang 42

M

Magnesium 59
and arrhythmias 51, 115
and tachycardia 88
Magnetic resonance imaging
(MRI) 95
Massage 100
for leg cramps 88
Meat 55
substituting 56
Meditation 104
Breathing 104
Humming 36
Mediterranean diet
and heart disease 56
Menopause
and heart disease 29
hormone replacement therapy
(HRT) 29
Minerals
as antioxidants 59
and fiber 60
for high blood pressure
125, 141
see also Magnesium,
Potassium
Myocardial infarction
see Heart attack
Myocardium 18

N

Natural therapies 98, 99
acupressure 101
acupuncture 101
aromatherapy 100
art therapy 149
autogenic training 42
biofeedback 104, 141
dance therapy 150
Feldenkrais Method 144
finding a therapist 100
herbal medicine 101
homeopathy 103
hydrotherapy 99, 122, 123
hypnotherapy 42, 104
massage 88, 100
meditation 36, 104
naturopathy 100, 122
traditional Chinese
medicine 101
yoga 104, 125, 151
Naturopathy 100, 122
Nervous system 21
and exercise 67
and smoking 34

O

Obesity
and blood pressure 51
and cholesterol 51
and diabetes 51
and heart disease 51
Oils 53, 57
fish 53
Oxygen 16
blood test for 91

P

Pacemakers 115
Palpitations 86, 87
and caffeine 64
ectopic heartbeat 88
see also Arrhythmias
Pericarditis 119
Pericardium 19
Personality
angry 152
types A, B 32, 152
Plaques 26
and age 26
and atherosclerosis 52
Positron emission tomography
(PET) scanning 95
Potassium 59
and arrhythmias 51, 115
and blood pressure reduction
51, 141
and tachycardia 88
Pregnancy
and blood pressure 41
and blood volume 25
Pulse 21
blood flow and 21
self-testing 97
in veins 90

R

Radionuclide tests 94
Rapid computed tomography
(CT) scanning 95
Relaxation
autogenic training 42
and blood pressure 82
combating disease with 82
flotation tank 83
herbs for 102
hydrotherapy for 99
massage for 100
at the office 148
and positive thinking 84
and sleep 132
technique 82
visualization 83
see also Stress relief
Risk factors for heart disease 28
avoidable 34
questionnaire 33

S

Salt (sodium)
and congestive heart
failure 121
and high blood pressure 51
substitutes 51
Saturated fats, in food 52
Second opinion 98
Senses, changes in 89
Sex, resuming after a heart
attack 137
Shock 89
Skin changes 89
Sleep, for heart patients 132
Smoking
and hyperlipoproteinemia
32
after a heart attack 137
and heart disease 28, 34
and intermittent claudication
129
passive, and heart disease 35
quitting 35
and weight gain 35
Sore throat
and valve infection 117
Stress
effects on heart and body 146
good and bad 40
and personality 40
reduction of 40
symptoms of 41
test (exercise ECG) 46
Stress relief 146
dance therapy for 150
herbs for 102
laughter 147
social support for 147
time management 148
yoga for 151
see also Relaxation
Stroke 127
art therapy 149
and aspirin 114
and atherosclerosis 108, 127
and blood pressure 41
brain hemorrhage 128
diet after 143
rehabilitation 128
Swollen ankles 86, 88

T

Thrombosis 125
and atherosclerosis 125
cerebral 128
coronary 126
deep vein 125
exercise for 127
and stroke 127
Traditional Chinese medicine 101
diagnosis in 93
Transplant, heart 119
Triglycerides
diet for lowering 143
and heart disease 29, 53

V

Valves 19
Valve disorders 115, 117
and arrhythmias 117
leaky (regurgitation) 115
replacement 118
stenosis 115
Valvuloplasty 118
Varicose veins 130
Veins 17
Ventricles 16, 19
Visualization 83, 137
for arteries 83
for quitting smoking 37
for relaxation 83
Vitamin
B and fetal heart rate 106
deficiency and heart muscle
disease 118, 119
see also Antioxidants

W

Weight
body mass index 51
chart, height/weight 97
control of 49, 143
daily calorie intake 53, 142
gain and smoking 35
obesity 51
pinch test 51
program for weight loss 74
see also Diet
Women
and heart disease 24, 29
see also Contraceptive pill,
Estrogen, Menopause,
Pregnancy

X

X-rays 94

Y

Yoga 104
breathing 104
for hypertension 125
for stress relief 151

Acknowledgments

Carroll & Brown Limited
would like to thank
Ellen Dupont
Sue Mimms
Garet Newell
Dr Mike Roth

British Heart Foundation

Tunturi Fitness Equipment supplied by
Bolton Stirland International Ltd.

Photograph sources

8 British Library, London/Bridgeman
Art Library, London
9 (Top) Zefa; (Bottom) Rex Features
10 Gordon White/photo courtesy of
Harefield Hospital patients
11 Robert Harding Picture Library/
Westlight International
12 Robert Harding Picture Library/
Sharpshooters
17 Professors P.M. Motta and
S. Correr/Science Photo Library
18 Royal College of Physicians,
London/Bridgeman Art Library,
London
21 Zefa
24 Zefa
32 Palazzo Corner Ca'Grande,
Venice/Bridgeman Art Library,
London
35 Zefa
39 Zefa
41 CNRI/Science Photo Library
42 (Top) Mary Evans Picture Library;
(Bottom) supplied by BAFATT
46 Tony Stone Images
84 Image Bank/Don King

93 Zefa
94 (Top) Science Photo Library;
(Centre) Science Photo Library;
(Bottom) Zefa
98 BSIP Ducloux/Science
Photo Library
99 Mary Evans Picture Library
101 Wellcome Institute Library,
London; (Right) Sally and
Richard Greenhill
104 Tony Stone Images
108 BSIP/Science Photo Library
110 Harry Smith Horticultural
Photographic Collection
115 Tony Stone Images
117 CNRI/Science Photo Library
118 Harry Smith Horticultural
Photographic Collection
120 News International/Rainbird
122 Mary Evans Picture Library
124 Stanford Eye Clinic/Science
Photo Library
126 (Top) Secchi-Lecaque/Roussel-
Uclaf/CNRI/Science Photo
Library; (Bottom) Professor P.M.
Motta/G. Macchiarelli/University
'La Sapienza', Rome/Science
Photo Library
128 (Top) Hattie Young/Science
Photo Library; (Bottom) Gca-
CNRI/Science Photo Library
129 Chris Bjornberg/Science
Photo Library
130 Zefa
137 Zefa
140 Zefa
144 Lionel Delevingne Photography
147 Zefa
150 Mary Evans Picture Library

Medical illustrators
Joanna Cameron
Richard Tibbitts

Illustrators
John Geary
Christine Pilsworth
Paul Williams
Angela Wood

Graphs
Nick Roland

Photographic assistants
Nick Allen
Sid Sideris

Hair and make-up
Rachel Attfield

Picture researcher
Sandra Schneider

Food preparation
Maddalena Bastianelli
Eric Treuille

Research
Laura Price

Index
Sharon Freed